Interdisciplinary Perspectives on Health Policy and Practice

For Churchill Livingstone:

Senior Commissioning Editor: Jacqueline Curthoys
Project Development Manager: Mairi McCubbin
Project Manager: Derek Robertson
Page Make-up: Gerard Heyburn

Interdisciplinary Perspectives on Health Policy and Practice

Competing interests or complementary interpretations?

Jane Robinson MA PhD MIPD RN ONC RHV HVT CertEd FRCN
Emeritus Professor, Postgraduate Division, School of Nursing,
University of Nottingham, Nottingham
Editor, Journal of Advanced Nursing

Mark Avis BA(Hons) MSc RMN RNT CertEd
Reader, School of Nursing,
University of Nottingham, Nottingham

Joanna Latimer BA(Hons) RN PhD
Research Officer in Social Gerontology, Centre for Social Gerontology,
Department of Applied Social Studies, Keele University, Keele

Michael Traynor MA(Cantab) PhD RN RHV
Lecturer, Centre for Policy in Nursing Research,
London School of Hygiene and Tropical Medicine, London

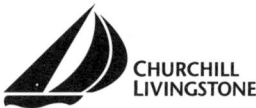

CHURCHILL LIVINGSTONE

EDINBURGH LONDON NEW YORK PHILADELPHIA ST LOUIS SYDNEY TORONTO TOK'

CHURCHILL LIVINGSTONE
An imprint of Harcourt Publishers Limited

First published 1999

ISBN 0 443 05992 6

British Library Cataloguing in Publication Data
A catalogue record for this book is available from the
British Library.

Library of Congress Cataloging in Publication Data
A catalog record for this book is available from the Library
of Congress.

The
publisher's
policy is to use
**paper manufactured
from sustainable forests**

Printed in China

Contents

Preface   vii

Introduction   1

1. Researching National Health Service reform in the 1980s: issues of substance and method   33
Jane Robinson

2. The World Bank and the World Health Organization: international sources of ideas for health policy   53
Jane Robinson

3. Health needs and health care needs   81
Mark Avis

4. Social justice and the right to health care   99
Mark Avis

5. Managers and measurement: taking a literary approach to managerial discourse   121
Michael Traynor

6. Morality and self-sacrifice in nursing talk   141
Michael Traynor

7. Interests and their realignment: managing medicine   163
Joanna Latimer

8. Interests and identity: nurses conducting care, performing disciplined subjects   185
Joanna Latimer

Epilogue   209

Index   213

Preface

Interdisciplinary Perspectives on Health Policy and Practice: competing interests or complementary interpretations? arose from a request to write a book on the politics of health care. The four authors had all been pursuing different aspects of this theme in their research since the late 1980s. From our many discussions it seemed that there was a place for a book which demonstrated some of the competing interests, and also the complementary perspectives, which exist across a range of practical situations in health care. *Interdisciplinary Perspectives on Health Policy and Practice* is not therefore an abstract treatise on the political science of health care but, instead, an account of our own research in the field, and some of the interpretations which we have drawn from it. That research is very diverse but our shared interest lies in developing an intellectual critique of contemporary health policy and practice. The Introduction sets that critique in the context of Edward Said's challenge to the contemporary intellectual to raise moral issues at the heart of even the most technical and professionalised activity. Said challenges us not to be afraid of confrontation and points out how, in an age of 'experts', it is very easy to be recruited to the dominant forces which shape every society. The introduction also includes our personal biographies written to explain our interest in the field of health care policy and practice, and some of the ideas and experiences which have shaped its development.

Two chapters written by each of the authors then follow. Jane Robinson first takes a retrospective and critical look at the research on the management of nursing following the Griffiths' reforms of the National Health Service which she carried out with Phil Strong during the second half of the 1980s at the University of Warwick. Her second chapter considers the ideas and events which have underpinned the historical development of the approaches to health care and health policy by the World Health Organization and The World

Bank. Drawing on both the historical literature and her own personal experience she concludes, tentatively, that as we approach the millenium there is some evidence of plurality rather than a polarisation of ideas.

Mark Avis's chapters draw on his philosophy training to consider the problems of meeting health needs and health care needs, and of social justice and the right to health care. In exploring the competing theoretical perspectives which tend to inform opposing positions on contemporary health policy and practice, Mark develops some of the philosophical arguments which underpin the practical dilemmas identified in the other six chapters. He concludes, drawing on Wittgenstein's Philosophical Investigations, that philosophy attempts to make sense of some of the profound questions about human life and how we should live. Hence, questions concerning the provision of health care need to be addressed through a continuing dialogue, for there is no 'right' way which is separate from our own endeavours to discover what is a good life, and how we should live it.

Michael Traynor describes how his dissatisfaction with the numerical aspects of a survey of job satisfaction amongst community nurses following the implementation of the Health Services and Community Care Act, 1990, led him back to the methods he had used as a student of literature. In treating the utterances of community nurses and their managers as 'text' he was able to engage in a discourse analysis which identified how their respective interests were constructed through the language they used and through appeals to more deep-seated structures of thought. In siding with neither nurses nor managers, Michael demonstrates how powerfully the values of a dominant discourse are played out through a duality of opposition with the discourse which is being subordinated.

Joanna Latimer's chapters also draw on empirical research which she carried out during the health care reforms of the early 1990s. Following older people and observing the delivery of their medical and nursing care when admitted to a prestigious teaching hospital, Joanna also assembled her field work material into a 'text'. She traced the way that these patients' identities were configured and re-configured in a range of situations. In trying to find theoretical explanations for the events which she observed, Joanna read and rejected many authors' views on the social processes in which the various actors engaged. Her account of how health care practitioners *themselves* define and account for their various behaviours shows just how subtly people's interests and identities become aligned with dominant values. This is no account of practitioners being 'forced' against their will to engage in unacceptable professional behaviours, but instead shows how easily they assume the values to which it is economically or politically expedient for them to aspire.

This then is a book which traces a number of political themes in contemporary health care policy and practice. It draws no final conclusions, for the four authors believe that the process of understanding and deciding upon the 'best' way is a continuous one. Maintaining that continuity of dialogue is a moral responsibility for each of us who, because we are social animals, must engage in this continuing discussion of how best competing interests and complementary perspectives should come together in the provision of health care.

In discussing acknowledgements we all agreed that first we should thank our respective families who, in the nature of writing books, provide so much invisible support and encouragement whilst we engage in this somewhat masochistic 'off duty' activity. Second, we thank Barbara Wade who directed the Daphne Heald Research Unit at the Royal College of Nursing and who supported Michael Traynor in the pursuit of this research, often by questioning his approach to data analysis. Third, we thank Anne-Marie Rafferty for her collegiality and friendship and for introducing Jane Robinson to the work of Edward Said. Jane Robinson also thanks the following: The Fulbright Commission of the United States of America for the award in 1997 of a Senior Research Scholarship which enabled her to spend three months with The World Bank in Washington DC and in Indonesia; staff in the Health, Nutrition and Population Sector of The World Bank for providing a unique learning experience during her visit; and staff of the World Health Organization for opportunities over a number of years to observe and to contribute to their work on nursing. Finally, we wish to acknowledge the support of each other in this enterprise. Our meetings and mutual discussions have been enriching and, as a result, the process has been very positive and remarkably trauma-free.

1999 JR, MA, JL, MT

Introduction

It is difficult when living through an era to step back and take a 'man from Mars' perspective on the key issues of the period. Nevertheless, investigative journalists and social researchers do this all the time by contributing critical commentary and interpretation to everyday events. As, in the United Kingdom at least, current debates on nursing education focus on its relevance to *practice*, it seems timely to consider nursing's ultimate intellectual and political development from a wider, critical perspective, and to show the potential contribution of different forms of analysis to such a project. In the present utilitarian age, when everything upon which money is spent has to be seen as having a direct relationship to an outcome of immediate *practical* importance, such a view may be seen as unfashionable. But writing *Interdisciplinary Perspectives on Health Policy and Practice: competing interests or complementary interpretations?*, undertaken in our own time and with no stronger motivation than to bring together some of the ideas with which our thinking as co-authors has been linked through numerous interpersonal encounters in research and teaching over the past decade, gave us the opportunity to cast our reflective net wider.

This is no self-indulgent reflection for, we believe, that such commentary has a crucial democratic role to play. The political deconstruction of nursing in relation to health care has, with a few notable exceptions, been largely invisible in terms of intellectual analysis. This is unacceptable for such a significant minority group whose contribution to health care, both in terms of its strengths *and* weaknesses, demands to be politically contextualised and better understood. Unfortunately, it is also unfashionable to declare oneself to be both a nurse *and* an intellectual. The two are generally seen to be mutually exclusive and incompatible. Yet, critical commentary on contemporary nursing is better informed if it is undertaken with a clear understanding both of the value systems of the intellectual, and with some personal experience and insight into actual health care practice.

Our personal credentials to undertake this ambitious task are set out in the second half of this introductory chapter. First, the notion of an intellectual critique is introduced. This section draws heavily on the clear exposition 'set out in the 1993 BBC Reith Lectures, *Representations of the Intellectual*, which were subsequently published under the same title (Said 1994). In this set of six lectures Edward Said reviewed much of the key literature on the subject and came to describe the essential role of contemporary intellectuals as providing critical, often unpopular, commentary on current states of affairs. Said's is a global perspective, written in terms of high politics, from the point of view of a Palestinian professor living and working in the United States of America (USA). Yet, virtually everything he says has resonances with writing critical commentary on nursing and health care, for he speaks of the intellectual's difficult task in analysing the position of the minority, the unrepresented, and the invisible, whilst standing personally between loneliness and alignment:

> There is no question in my mind that the intellectual belongs on the same side with the weak and unrepresented. Robin Hood some are likely to say. Yet it's not that simple a role, and therefore cannot easily be dismissed as just so much romantic idealism. At bottom, the intellectual, in my sense of the word, is neither a pacifier nor a consensus builder, but someone whose whole being is staked on a critical sense, a sense of being unwilling to accept easy formulas, or ready made cliches, or the smooth ever so accommodating confirmations of what the powerful or conventional have to say, and what they do. Not just passively unwilling, but actively willing to say so in public.
>
> (Said 1994, pp. 22–23)

Said describes the 20th century as an era with a general group of men and women called intellectuals or the intelligentsia. Unlike the 19th century, when intellectuals tended to be solitary rather aloof, nonconforming creatures who were frequently seen as rebels against established opinion, the intellectuals of the 20th century are paid for their opinions in jobs such as management, universities, journalists or government experts. This is, after all, the age of the 'expert' society. Said wonders whether, as a result, the independent voice of the individual intellectual can exist at all in the 20th century outside some closeted existence where contact with, and commentary on, the real world is tenuous and muted (Said 1994, pp. 65–83). Yet for Said, critical commentary must be contextualised directly with the events of the 'real' world despite all the personal risks of loneliness and alienation.

Said's viewpoint has tremendous resonance with people working in 20th century health care, where there is only the finest of dividing lines between the responses to critical intellectual commentary of those in power and their reactions to 'whistle blowing' activities by staff. Opposition to these forms of challenge rarely manifests itself in direct action, but the British establishment has powerful, if subtle, ways of silencing those who believe that it is legitimate in their role to speak out critically on the perceived deficits in *any* situation. Said's answer is for the intellectual to be an amateur:

> someone who considers that to be a thinking and concerned member of a society one is entitled to raise moral issues at the heart of even the most technical and professionalized activity as it involves one's country, its power, its mode of interacting with its citizens as well as other societies. In addition, the intellectual's spirit as an amateur can enter and transform the merely professional routine most of us go through into something more lively and radical; instead of doing what one is supposed to do one can ask why one does it, who benefits from it, how it can reconnect with a personal project and original thoughts.
>
> (Said 1994, p. 83)

For Said, nothing is more reprehensible than the actions of the intellectual which induce avoidance of confrontation with a position which one knows to be morally unprincipled. Said may have in mind the actors in an international political community when he writes the following, but its resonance will be felt by many who work in contemporary universities, or health care:

> You do not want to appear too political; you are afraid of appearing controversial; you need the approval of the boss or an authority figure; you want to keep a reputation for being balanced, objective, moderate; your hope is to be asked back, to consult, to be on a board or prestigious committee, and so to remain within the responsible mainstream; some day you hope to get an honorary degree, a big prize, perhaps even an ambassadorship.
>
> (Said 1994, p. 101)

Said's solution to these peculiarly 20th century dilemmas is to speak truth to power; to weigh the alternatives, picking the right one and representing it where it can do most good. As he so eloquently describes from a global political perspective, this is no easy task. It is one which must be learned painfully, often in isolation from one's peers. Yet if, as nursing education enters the universities, it is to begin to take on the mantle of the intellectual it is precisely these matters which must be addressed. The debates concerning whether such transitions are about the ascendancy of academia over practice are sterile and self-defeating. As Said shows, intellectual critique cannot *exist* without practice. It is how these critiques are developed, theoretically justified, and transmuted into action that matters. It is from this perspective that this book is written.

As the four authors, we have each in previous respective researches contributed analysis and commentary, written mainly although not exclusively with a focus on nursing, on the ways in which political and socioeconomic forces have impacted on health care development during the 1980s and 1990s. In *Interdisciplinary Perspectives on Health Policy and Practice: competing interests or complementary interpretations?* we bring independent perspectives to bear on the subject matter of our individual chapters, but we share the underlying theme of an intellectual critique.

This does not mean that we share a single methodological orientation, but instead share a concern to understand and explain the tensions experienced by many of those working in contemporary health care. These tensions arise on the one hand from a utilitarian rationality, driven by governments under financial constraint and frequently critical of traditional welfare notions and, on the other, the often explicitly moral orientation expressed by nurses. Further, these tensions, whilst researched frequently in the micro-context of a local health care setting, are apparently ubiquitous throughout the world irrespective of geography, political government or national economic situation. In particular, nursing is forced increasingly to represent its activities in terms of a managerialist discourse, and alternative discourses such as a moral self-representation are becoming 'disqualified' and less easy to maintain.

The *'competing interests'* of the subtitle can therefore be interpreted in two ways. First, we examine the competing interests of the various actors in the theatre of health care. We look at issues not simply as a matter of competition for power and control but also how these concepts are *constructed* through various *behavioural devices* which can be *deconstructed* theoretically. Forms of *language* have an important role here. Second, the origins of the different *ideological perspectives* subscribed to by the various actors in health care, and which underpin the observed behaviour, can also be seen as competing and capable of *deconstruction*. *Utilitarian versus deontological* philosophical perspectives have an important place here. The *complementary interpretations* of the subtitle refers to the ways in which ideas rarely remain polarised at one or other end of a continuum. When analysing the *policy process* it is frequently the case that in its *application* key actors can be seen to be mediating and shifting between positions which at first sight appear irreconcilable.

NURSES' DEVELOPING POLITICAL AWARENESS

Interdisciplinary Perspectives on Health Policy and Practice: competing interests or complementary interpretations? would appear to be timely, for a notable feature of the history of British nursing during the last two decades of this century has been an increasing political awareness amongst nurses. This development has been demonstrated in three interlinked strands. First, growing political awareness has been reflected in a number of publications on the politics of nursing emerging during the period (Clay 1987, Robinson 1991, Robinson et al 1992, Salvage 1985, Strong & Robinson 1990, White 1985, 1986, 1988). Further, perhaps partly as a result of these publications, nurses are increasingly confident in including political perspectives in contemporary research and publications.

Second, growing political astuteness has been shown by many leaders of nursing in their dealings with government. Unfortunately, much of this activity remains hidden from the public world view of nurses. Yet, an example of nursing's expanding influence in government circles may be seen from the growth during the 1990s in nursing research activities, an unprecedented growth which might have been thought impossible less than a decade ago. Of course, there is still a long way to go and many factors have undoubtedly led to this state of affairs, nevertheless the roles of the professional organisations, and of nurses working in government as civil servants have undoubtedly played a substantial part. Third, the multidisciplinary forms of higher education to which many nurses have subscribed, partly through choice, partly through necessity in the absence of many centres of nursing in higher education, has led some nursing commentators to develop alternative theoretical *explanations* rather than mere *descriptions* of social and political phenomena in health care.

A related but notable recent development, The Royal College of Nursing's (RCN) Association of Nursing Students' Resolution to the 1997 RCN Congress, 'That this meeting of the RCN Congress supports the introduction of political education as an integral part of pre-registration courses' (RCN 1997), demonstrates not only a growing awareness, but also a need for political education even at the level of pre-registration.

The personal encounters which have given rise to our collaboration in writing this book have been made possible by an expanding intellectual infrastructure arising from the incorporation of nursing into higher education, and the burgeoning of research on nursing and health care already mentioned. This has led to increased self-confidence in sharing ideas and writing on political issues. It is perhaps worth reflecting that, although natural to be preoccupied with the search for resources for nursing *practice*, it is also easy to overlook the huge benefits of this crucially important development of a 'critical mass' of social and political commentators on nursing issues.

British nursing has had both advantages and disadvantages arising from this relatively late development of political awareness. For example, unlike their British counterparts, nurses in the USA had a head start in political emancipation during the early years of the 20th century. Davies (1980) in a comparative study of British and North American nursing from the beginning of the 20th century to 1939, suggests that, in part, this may be explained by the fact that North American nurses had far greater confidence than their British counterparts. The USA at the beginning of this century was a relatively 'new' country where the emancipation of women's work (including nursing) may have been a necessary factor in the building of both a national identity and an economic infrastructure. Meritocracy at the beginning of the 20th century was not so much an ideology in the USA as an economic necessity. Davies suggests therefore that the defining and achieving of nursing's policy goals cannot be understood as divorced from the cultural context in which they are formulated. There were differences in the American legislative framework, patterns of employment for nurses and, crucially, the educational system where nursing was well established in some universities from before the Second World War.

Britain, by contrast, was a deeply paternalistic, class-based, colonial power. Florence Nightingale, the nurse selected by the 'great and the good' of the British establishment to epitomise everything desirable in British nurses, preferred a structure for nursing based on the class system of which she was so firmly a part (Rafferty 1996).

As a result, higher education for nurses in Britain was seen at the beginning of the 20th century to be unnecessary for the 'ordinary' practitioner who would always be bound by the orders of either her superintendent, or a member of the medical profession. Hardy (1986) and Simnett (1986) have both demonstrated the subtle ways in which class and gender have interacted historically in British nursing.

British nurses who wished therefore to be a part of an intellectual endeavour had to look to disciplines outside nursing in order to develop their theoretical frameworks. Many of these were in the humanities or social sciences which, by their nature, encouraged nurses to take a critical view of the subject matter of nursing and health care. This, we would argue has produced, almost by default, one of the *advantages* of the late development in British nurses' political awareness. Instead of being 'locked in' to a 'monotechnic' educational environment where the sole focus of concern was the 'here and now' of nursing practice, British nurses who have ventured into the wider fields of intellectual endeavour have been encouraged to set the phenomena of 'practice' in far wider frameworks for understanding and explanation.

It is from this critical academic tradition that the four authors of *Interdisciplinary Perspectives on Health Policy and Practice: competing interests or complementary interpretations?* originate. It is no surprise that Joanna Latimer and Michael Traynor, with their interests in the analysis of discourses employed in health care practices, should have both read English at university before becoming nurses; or that Mark Avis, with his interest in human need and equity, should have read Philosophy after becoming a mental health nurse. My own decision to pursue Master's and PhD degrees in a Department of Sociology, Social Anthropology and Social Policy arose initially from my dissatisfaction with the official explanations offered in the 1970s for the lack of interprofessional communication in child abuse cases. This, in turn, led to a widening interest in the diverse ways in which power and control are exercised in health and social care, and in the ways in which they may be studied.

As a result of this experience, it has always appeared to me as a teacher and researcher, that nurses have a tremendous amount both to give to, and to take from, academic disciplines which at first sight may appear to have relatively little to do with nursing practice. The insights which emerge from these forms of intellectual activity are not, however, always comfortable to live with. 'Critical' intellectual disciplines constantly challenge 'received wisdom' and the 'status quo'. It is therefore appropriate to reflect that as *Interdisciplinary Perspectives on Health Policy and Practice: competing interests or complementary interpretations?* was being written, the wholesale move of British nursing into higher education offered highly relevant intellectual opportunities which may at first sight have little to do with nursing practice. Once taken up and understood, however, they offer a significant means for nurses to understand both just how much needs to be done, and the very real constraints in trying to achieve lasting and effective change in nursing practice.

OUR PERSONAL BIOGRAPHIES

Impersonal theoretical accounts of a particular 'reality' tend to be a feature of traditional academic writing. Apart from a brief, highly selective vignette on the back cover of a book it is not usually expected that the reader needs to know anything more about an author. This totally impersonal style is closely linked to modernism and the rise of scientific inquiry. The text is seen to be sufficient in itself. An alternative view is that as the text conveys a particular construction of reality, the reader needs to know from which personal orientation the author comes. This is particularly the case when writing about power and control, and various forms of oppression. It is a view which lies at the heart of the feminist perspective that 'the personal is political' and Edward Said, quoted extensively above, believes strongly that the contemporary context of a situation must be understood in order for genuine critical analysis to take place. We arrived at a decision therefore that our introduction would include an account from each of us which would explain how our situation in nursing scholarship arose, and why we took the particular approach we did to the subject matter of our chapters. These now follow in the alphabetical order of the authors' names.

Mark Avis

In 1981 I qualified as a Registered Mental Nurse and, during my first year working on an acute admission ward, began to develop what was to become an abiding interest in philosophy. Sparked off by concern about the nature of rationality and the ethics of compulsory detention in hospital I began reading introductory texts on philosophy. I was mystified but curious that philosophy, as a subject, did not seem to offer ready answers to moral questions about rationality, rights or paternalism. Instead philosophy offered a discursive narrative of ideas, an ebb and flow of argument and counter-argument, in response to fundamental questions about human life. Many of these enquiries had their origins in the classical period of Ancient Greece. However, my desire to study the subject was kindled by the conviction in philosophy that arguing about ideas does matter, that ideas make a difference. The next year, in 1982, I started a full-time philosophy degree at King's College, London. I was fortunate to study under Professor Peter Winch, whose book *The Idea of a Social Science* (Winch 1958) on the application of Wittgenstein's ideas about the social significance of rule-following as a way of understanding language and culture had become influential in social sciences.

After completing my degree, I returned to nursing but continued to think and read about philosophical issues. I eventually arrived in the Department of Nursing Studies at the University of Nottingham where Jane Robinson was Professor and Head of Department. Jane was, and remains, committed to the notion that, although nursing is an intensely practical activity, abstract ideas do matter. She nurtured my interest in applying philosophical analysis to the subject and the discipline of nursing enquiry. The direction that this interest took was in examining the epistemological basis of qualitative nursing enquiry. It appeared that the debate in the nursing and social science literature had shown a tendency to degenerate into lists of polarised attributes. We have been given positivism versus anti-positivism; absolutism versus relativism; quantitative versus qualitative paradigms; science versus deconstruction; objective versus subjective, facts versus values, and so on. As such, it appeared to me that this debate had more to do with rhetoric than philosophical analysis. The role that philosophy was playing in this debate was to provide an epistemological foundation for theoretical or methodological perspectives. I think that the danger inherent in this use of philosophy is that it strips philosophical arguments from their place in the historical narrative of ideas in order to justify a particular point of view. This error is exemplified by the use of phenomenology in some qualitative nursing research methodologies (Paley 1997). An opposing danger comes when philosophy is used to argue that there are *no* foundations for any enquiry, that everything is relative. I believe that Wittgenstein's *Philosophical Investigations* (1953) suggests a way of thinking about the application of philosophy that avoids the idea that philosophy can be used to provide a secure foundation for academic enquiry. Instead, he offers a view of philosophy as an attempt to make sense of some questions about human life, who we are and how we should live, and, most important of all, how to make the results of these enquiries intelligible.

Chapters 3 and 4 are based on this alternative view of philosophy. These chapters pose two questions: whether people have real, objective health needs; and whether as a society we ought to help people meet some of their health needs. These would appear to be two quite distinct questions. The former asks as a matter of *fact* whether people have universal and objective health needs, the latter asks whether we have a *duty* to assist people who are unable to meet their own health needs. It would seem that the first question should be settled by scientific enquiry, the second by ethical analysis. However, this is to see the pursuit of knowledge about who we are and how we should live as conceptually distinct enquiries, a formulation that would be completely alien to a classical philosopher such as Aristotle. It is to be in the grip of a view about knowledge which sees scientific enquiry as answering questions about matters of fact; and discards what cannot be answered through the application of science as mere subjective opinion or dogma. Any academic pursuit that does not use the scientific method is therefore dismissed as engaging in rhetoric. Michael Traynor touches on this issue in his introduction where he acknowledges the influence that philosophers such as Richard Rorty and Michel Foucault have had on his approach to academic enquiry. In particular, Michael notes their attempts to deal with the problem of knowledge and present a picture of enquiry that is consistent with the diversity of academic practices and accepts the fallibility of all human pursuits.

This fits with my own view that the most profound puzzles in philosophy are given by the relation between human culture, invention, and a conception of an objective world beyond human experience. The common metaphors that we use to explain the nature of 'objective knowledge' contain a relational element; we often say that our beliefs or statements are true when they *correspond* to reality or *mirror* 'how the world is'. On reflection, it should be obvious that the only way we can find out 'how the world is' is through the processes of human experience and invention. The mutual interdependence of truth, reality and human invention would seem to contradict these simple relational metaphors. How can we check whether our beliefs and statements correspond to 'how the world is' except through the application of our limited and all too fallible human faculties? We appear to be caught in an epistemological trap that blurs the distinction between human invention and 'how the world is', and undermines any certainty that we can have objective knowledge about 'how the world is'.

This gap between our epistemological metaphors, our aspirations for objective knowledge, and our limited and fallible powers of human perception is exploited by the sceptic. The sceptic shows that we never have sufficient evidence to support our claims to know what is real and true, and that doubt will always undermine any claim to knowledge. The modern form of the profound sceptic is provided by Descartes in his influential 'Meditations' (1637). He imagines that everything that he perceives could be the result of the machinations of an 'evil demon' who systematically deceives him about what is real and what is an illusion. This version of the profound sceptic has been updated by Putnam who creates a thought experiment in which we could all be 'brains in a vat' connected to a giant computer which generates all our perceptions (Putnam 1981). These versions of the epistemological sceptic undermine any faith that we can have certain knowledge about 'how the world is'.

One way of responding to the sceptic is to find some secure foundation for knowledge that insulates us from doubt. Descartes, using his famous formulation, *cogito ergo sum* (I think therefore I am), attempted to find an epistemological principle about which he could not be deceived which would then allow him to find a basis for certain knowledge. An alternative approach is to argue that science is just such a foundational activity. In this light, the phenomenal success of science during the past 500 years would seem to be a practical response to the sceptic. Science provides a way of obtaining a view of the world that gives us objective knowledge freed from our contingent and subjective human experiences.

It is common practice to associate the rising tide of science during the last half of the millennium with the 'enlightenment project'. This is summarised succinctly by Luntley (1995) as 'the project to attain the truth that is available from the God's eye point of view, the truth that makes up the grand narrative about the whole of creation' (pp. 11–12). He goes on to argue that modernists secularised the enlightenment project and removed the idea of God from the account. The modernists' objective is to tell the 'world's own story', and they believe that the scientific method is the instrument with which to write the world's own story. In so far as it is intelligible to talk about the 'enlightenment project', philosophers have sometimes seen their role as elucidating the foundational language with which to tell the world's own story. 17th and 18th century empiricist philosophers such as Locke and Hume saw themselves as clarifying the relation between human thought and the world and, to simplify greatly, modernist philosophers have shifted their attention to the relation between language and the world. In this century positivist philosophers and scientists such as Mach, Ayer and Carnap thought that the language of logic and mathematics would provide the medium with which to tell the 'world's own story'.

What disturbs me about this view of science as a foundation for epistemology is that it appears to relegate philosophy to a marginal role in the quest for knowledge. Peter Winch (1958) terms it the 'underlabourer conception of philosophy'. He quotes Locke's introduction to his *Essay Concerning Human Understanding* (Locke 1964) to summarise this point of view, 'In advancing the sciences ... it is ambition enough to be employed as an under-labourer in clearing the ground a little, and removing some of the rubbish that lies in the way to knowledge' (p. 58). On this view, the path to knowledge is laid through the application of the scientific method, and philosophy provides the analytical tools to resolve any linguistic tangles that obstruct the path. Winch (1958) argues that these tangles are largely conceived of as arising from anomalies in the use and application of our all too human language, and rather like a mechanic, 'a philosopher removes contradictions from the realms of discourse' (p. 5).

I find myself in sympathy with many postmodernist philosophers, such as Rorty, because they reject the underlabourer conception of philosophy and try to rehabilitate philosophical enquiry (Rorty 1991). They also repudiate the modernist confidence that science will be able to tell us the story of the world from the point of view of the universe. Postmodernists, like latter-day sceptics, exploit the gap between our metaphors and our aspirations about objective knowledge, and provide us with good reason to doubt the ability of science to tell the 'world's own story'. Their arguments draw on some well-known philosophical problems of empirical science that have been identified during the past 40 years (Davidson 1984, Goodman 1983, Quine 1960, Van Fraassen 1980). They point out that there is never sufficient empirical evidence to support any epistemological claim with certainty; we can always turn out to have been mistaken. Furthermore, they point out that all empirical evidence is theory dependent; even something as simple as taking a reading from a thermometer depends upon theories of optics and thermodynamics. The theory dependence of all empirical evidence undermines a foundationalist view of scientific knowledge. Postmodernists also draw on Kuhn's historical analysis of science which shows that the advancement of knowledge is not a smooth and steady progress towards 'objective knowledge' (Kuhn 1970). On the contrary, Kuhn describes how the growth of scientific knowledge is more like a series of arbitrary 'paradigm shifts' and 'gestalt switches'. Postmodernists support this observation by drawing upon examples given by sociologists of science, who demonstrate that scientific practice is both contingent and non-rational (Barnes & Edge 1982). They argue that the social institution of science publicly espouses the values of objective enquiry but operates so as to maintain authority in the production of knowledge.

Rorty's postmodern spin on the problems of empirical science provides a good reason to doubt the foundational view of science (Rorty 1991). For if scientific enquiry does not define the nature of objective knowledge, then other academic enquiries which aspire to produce knowledge are released from the need to ape its methods. Indeed, it is the idea of science as foundational that, as Rorty points out, divides our intellectual heritage into series of unwelcome antitheses: fact and value; objective and subjective; and truth and opinion. His version of postmodernism offers an analysis of knowledge that relieves science of its special status and resolves some these dichotomies. However, many of those who follow a postmodernist line of argument have gone on to argue that if science is not a foundation for objective knowledge then there can be no objective knowledge at all (Lyotard 1985). In a sense this is the old sceptical argument in a bright new postmodern garb. If science does not define the nature of objective knowledge, then all knowledge is contingent, culturally and historically specific, and discourse dependent. The only criteria for the acceptability of knowledge are internal to each type of academic enquiry, and since these criteria are specific to each discipline and incommensurate with each other then we must draw a conclusion of epistemological relativism with regard to academic enquiry. It seems important to reject this epistemological relativism for two reasons. First, it devalues one of the principal virtues of academic enquiry which is to engage in critical dialogues. Second, anti-foundationalism rests on the mistaken assumption that objective knowledge requires a non-temporal, non-contextual and ahistorical point of view with which to make a judgement about a claim of knowledge. In this sense relativists are victims of the view they deconstruct. It places the conduct of human enquiry in a false dilemma; either to allow standards of objectivity that are acultural and ahistorical or to accept that all enquiry is perspectival, culturally and historically conditioned.

I want to offer a view of philosophy, science and academic enquiry that accepts the postmodern critique of science but which avoids anti-foundationalism and epistemological relativism. Winch (1958) offers a second version of the relationship between philosophy and science as an alternative to the underlabourer conception of philosophy. It is a conception of philosophy as a *therapeutic* activity. Philosophy concerns an elucidation of the conditions that make reality *intelligible* to us in our shared cultural life. Winch argues that:

> To ask whether reality is intelligible is to ask about the relation between thought and reality. In considering the nature of thought one is led also to consider the nature of language. Inseparably bound up with the question of whether reality is intelligible, therefore, is the question of how language is connected with reality, of what it is to *say* something.

(Winch 1958, pp. 11–12)

This view of philosophy calls into question the construction of the sceptical argument. It holds that it cannot *make sense* to believe that knowledge depends upon taking a view of the world that transcends human capabilities. Whatever we may mean by 'objective knowledge', human experience is all we have, and knowledge about 'how the world is' must be attained and checked through the application of human reason and systematic human enquiry. Science may be one of the most successful academic enquiries, but it does not, and cannot, give a view of the world that transcends the human perspective. A holistic view of epistemology, drawing upon the therapeutic conception of philosophy, can help us here. This version of epistemology does not try to identify a foundation for all knowledge, instead it maintains that knowledge depends upon how different academic enquiries interlock. The most appropriate metaphor is that knowledge is like a boat at sea. Although the boat is not in direct contact with an epistemological foundation of dry land, its ability to stay afloat derives from the interconnectedness of its planks. Human knowledge draws its strength from the bonds that can be formed between academic enquiries. However, like in a boat, none of the planks that make up human knowledge is irreplaceable, and any one of them may be changed for another if the new plank fits better than the old, just so long as we do not attempt to change all of the planks at the same time! A holistic view of knowledge changes our idea of objectivity. Objectivity is concerned with obtaining the best available human perspective rather than an attempt to take the point of view of the universe. Objectivity is not about trumping all other points of view; it arises out a search for consensus, for a better fitting of the planks of knowledge through seeking out dialogue between enquiries.

Why dialogue matters

Rorty (1991) argues that the desire for objectivity 'boils down to a desire to acquire beliefs which will eventually receive unforced agreement in the course of free and open encounter with people holding other beliefs' (p. 41). The implication is that dialogue between discourses is not only possible, but that achieving rational consensus through dialogue is the object of human enquiry, and the ideal of objectivity. This pragmatic criterion would allow that facts and knowledge can be both objective and contested. Rorty argues that points of disagreement between enquiries are resolved by trying to 'weave them together with beliefs we already have' (p. 38), a metaphor that Quine (1980) has also used: 'our vaguely pragmatic inclination to adjust one strand in the fabric of science rather than another in accommodating some particularly recalcitrant experience' (p. 46). This interlocking metaphor for knowledge is a coherent alternative to the image of correspondence or mirroring. We do not have to give up ideas of objectivity, or treat objective facts with scepticism, or allow that where there are conflicting discourses there is judgemental relativism with no hope of settling the matter. On the contrary, it would seem that rational dispute in search of unforced agreement is a defining feature of objectivity. This allows an Aristotelian notion of academic pursuit that does not separate enquiries into facts and values, science and opinion, or detach an understanding of what we are from how we should live. Our shared intellectual tradition provides us with enough resources, values, beliefs and practices to allow a certain degree of dialogue about the kind of society we live in and kind of society we ought to have. The debate about health care need and social justice would seem to be part of this dialogue.

Joanna Latimer: my story, or the continuing translation of my interests!

Having read English Literature at the University of London, I worked in a rural hospital for elderly people, as a cleaner and then as a nursing auxiliary. I was continuously shocked by the plight of the older people in this hospital. It was the district dumping ground, nursing practice was routinised and hierarchical, and patients were treated as if they were stabled. But the facilities were clean and fresh, with good equipment, a veranda and sitting rooms, and the food was all home cooked. Matron lived in the residential half of the institution: she never seemed to do much at all, but smelt of alcohol. The consultant geriatrician would come once a week, when we all had to wait in the sluice, forbidden to undertake any nursing care during his round. We changed all the incontinent patients before his arrival, because, Sister said, he would not examine them if they were soiled. The nurses were mainly auxiliaries and enrolled nurses (ENs), there were two part-time Sisters, who seemed to have very little influence over the ENs and auxiliaries. Auxiliaries had a lot of responsibility: they might be on their own for part of a shift, they often helped to do the drug round.

When we came on in the mornings we gave everyone breakfast, then we would sit in the bathrooms, smoking and drinking tea. After this first break we would put those people who should have their bowels open on commodes, in the middle of the ward, with no screens around them. Some of us would make the beds, 38 of them on each floor. There was a bath book and everyone got a bath once a week; otherwise they were washed and dressed and sat in their chairs, or were kept in bed if they had too many contractures to be able to sit in a chair. Some patients were independent and did these things for themselves. All dependent patients were given endless pressure area care, no one had a pressure sore. Some of the patients were considered senile, some ranted and raved. Disruptive patients were told off: 'Oh Annie, you still haven't had your bowels open', as Annie was hoisted off the commode after 20 minutes, by two of us both peering into the pot; 'Umf, you are so heavy', as Annie was released back down onto the pot for another 10 minutes. The cleaners were very kind, it was they who knew many of the patients as many of them were farmers' and farm workers' wives, and the patients were mainly farmers, farm workers or local people. Families came at visiting time: patients on the whole seemed to be, and some seemed to feel, abandoned. I can remember the rituals over death: laying someone out, tying up his penis with a cotton bandage with a bow, stuffing his bottom with cotton wool. Everything dirty was to be continuously tidied up, anything disordering kept within bounds. Interestingly, the positive things about the hospital (its spotlessness, and freshness, the pressure areas, keeping the patients clean and nice to look at) seemed to all be being done with visitors or the staff themselves in mind. I cannot remember anyone, apart from the cleaners, saying that we should be doing things with the patients' concerns in mind.

I used to make drawings of the patients, and talk to them. I loved and pitied many of these people, and I wanted to do it better, find a way to understand, and change it.

So I subsequently trained as a nurse at University College Hospital (UCH). My training at UCH helped me to maintain some notion that patients were people, and that conduct, and the social life of patients *and* nurses is as important as all the technical prowess in the world. Bernie, a nursing officer in ICU, said to me one night: 'A chimpanzee can be trained to look after a ventilator, but not the person on the end of it'. My memories of my training are that it was full of emotion, an intensity of emotion. I was allowed to do something with all this emotion, because the hospital had an ethos of patient-centredness, something intangible, but always present: at handovers Sisters listened to you and explained the reasons for things, on ward rounds doctors listened to Sisters, and at the bedside, doctors and nurses listened to patients and watched them carefully. Not always, but a lot of the time. And it mattered how you were in the world: not just how you looked, but how you conducted yourself, and this was always accounted for as important because it was to do with how patients saw you. Early on, a Sister said to us, 'If you come on in the morning bedraggled, as if you cannot look after yourself, how will the patients or their families think you can look after them?' You were kept on your toes because you must always keep patients in mind. I remember wanting to do everything perfectly, as if I was always being watched, making a good impression. In school, when things were going badly, when the gap between being perfect and practice seemed to yawn wider, we were frustrated. The tutors listened to you, and one, Judy Muir, would always ask me when I was full of criticism, 'So, Joanna, how will you do it when *you* are in charge?' We had many deprived patients, tramps, and alcoholics, drug addicts and so forth, but they were included; even the accident and emergency department had been designed and built to take account of these people: every night there were homeless people sleeping on the floor of the outpatient section.

Institutions, then, not just individuals, have a life, they are a language, a continuous speaking of the things which matter, which must be made to count. Later I staffed in a surgical and radiotherapy ward. Then I helped to set up an innovatory unit: the first inner-city GP community hospital. I had joint responsibility for shaping this as a nurse-led, practice development unit which aimed at being research-driven. This was tough, getting ourselves to let go of the old boundaries, the old defences; but the senior nurses were good, they supported us, they were innovatory and had a real eye on possibilities for change. I then returned to acute nursing, and used my experience and understandings of community nursing, multidisciplinary liaison and research, to inform the reshaping of patient assessment and care in a medical ward environment. I tried to make it patient and family centred. This was not so easy: there were hierarchies and layers of stuff getting in the way, the hospital just was not patient focused, something was out of balance, it was too academic, too medically oriented, too formal. Importantly, though, it was here that I was reminded of my early experiences: older people were cared for but they were not wanted, they were regarded as getting in the way. What struck me was how I was continually reminded that what I wanted to do, for example getting families involved in care, was good but not appropriate to an acute environment. I took no notice and did it anyway, but I realised that here was a 'false' division that had something to do with time: for the hospital there was a focus on speed, and disposal, while for many of our patients illness was going to be with them for a long time (they had leukaemia or lymphoma, or a stroke):

they had illnesses which went on and on, reverberating on through their and their families' lives.

I won a Scottish Home and Health Department Nursing Research Training Fellowship. My subsequent doctoral education at the University of Edinburgh was as a social scientist. My PhD focused on the problem of bed-blocking, and the assessment and care of older people in acute medical contexts. To examine assessment of older people, I chose to do an ethnographic study in an acute medical unit (as my own field of expertise), and to focus on the assessment and care of 20 older patients, because I felt that ill older people needed to have good, patient-centred assessment if their futures were to be managed and supported appropriately. I believed that by following *patients* through a hospital unit, rather than staff, from their admission to their discharge or death, I could trace and show the ways in which nurses' practised nursing assessment, and how these practices related to the practices of others, to doctors and the patients themselves. So I located myself at the bedside of patients, and observed all their encounters with nurses and others. But I also travelled with patients on their journeys (for example to the bathroom, on home assessments) and through their stories of their everyday lives, their illness and their time in hospital. I also travelled with nurses' and others' representations of patients (for example, patients' profiles, stories of observation, temperature charts) on their journeys (through nurses' handovers, ward rounds, case conferences, in-patient documents, GP's letters). I watched what people did, and I listened to people. I was particularly interested in hearing people talk to each other, and give each other accounts of what they were doing, or of what they understood to be the problems and needs of patients. I also talked to people: to patients and nurses, and others, about their work, their illnesses, their lives, how they felt about themselves and their futures.

All field material was assembled into a 'text' (Latimer 1998a,b, Silverman 1987, 1993). The text was analysed using a constant comparative method (see Baruch 1981, cited in Silverman 1993), which drew on aspects of anthropological (Fernandez 1986a,b, Marcus & Fischer 1986, Strathern 1991, 1992, 1994, 1995, Turner 1967, Tyler 1986) discourse (Fairclough 1992, 1993, Silverman 1987, 1993) and conversation analysis (Silverman 1993, 1997). Analysis of field material as a text allowed me to trace the ways in which different patients' identities were being configured, both over time, and across interactions, in different registers (written, verbal, electrocardiographic, thermometric, radiographic, etc.), in different locations and by different assemblages of people and things.

My theoretical enlightenment occurred as I did the study and particularly during the analysis of research material. I read widely in contemporary social theory, but the main influences came from Foucault on the one hand, and the early ethnomethodologists, such as Bittner, Garfinkel and Sudnow, on the other. Later, in the writing of the study I have drawn more and more on contemporary anthropologists. My interest is the relationship between the conduct of social actors, considered as the intersection between disciplinary knowledge (e.g. management, nursing, medicine), the politics of distribution and identity. In analysing the research material I felt that there must be a way of understanding this relationship which did not just normalise: I was frustrated by nursing theory which constantly criticised practice, reiterating over and over that nurses *'need'* to do this because patient's *'need'* to have that. Writing which turned people either into romantic heroes or conspiratorial power freaks seemed to allow ideology to get in the way of analytical rigour. Nor did the structuralists satisfy me with ideas that we are just socialised, programmed, Garfinkel's (1967) cultural dopes, who do what they do because of their class, gender or ethnic origins. I wanted, like other writers that I admire, to exercise a more 'capacious soul': not just to point the finger, but develop a rigour to my work by not just putting practitioners or some other group down, to offer recommendations and solutions to the problems with their practice which I had managed to define for them; neither did I want to privilege myself as able to speak on anyone else's behalf. Following the practices of the ethnomethodologists, my concern is to reflect the complexity and fluidity of everyday life, and, following Foucault, at the same time understand why practitioners might be doing these things rather than those things; that is, how and why some relations or processes seem to reappear, over and over again. So while my central concern is power relations, this is not just to do with domination, but with how things get organised the ways that they do, how people and things get moved around or positioned to speak or act in these ways, rather than those ways, and what the effects of these ways of speaking and acting may accomplish, rather than those. So the concern is for what is made present and what is made absent, and the *play* of difference.

I have increasingly developed a style of analysis which pushes back cause and effect relations, although I am very interested in how others attribute an effect with a cause, to consider the conditions under which some effects are possible. This style attempts to treat all activities (policy documents, nursing at the bedside, accounting, statistical analyses, writing a book) as practices and as cultural artefacts. Rather than privilege one set of practices over another, or one kind of knowledge over another, I examine *how* practitioners themselves (such as policy makers, nurses, accountants, statisticians, authors, patients) privilege and account for their and others' conduct, their or others' knowledge, or one kind of evidence rather than another. Critically I explore what it is that they might be accomplishing by their methods, and how these methods are locating them in sociocultural time and space.

In summary then, the methodological approach taken in the study which I draw on in Chapters 7 and 8 focused on the distinctions which nurses and other professional carers put into play to figure the identities of people as patients with needs. Rather than considering these distinctions as 'givens', as matters of expert interpretation, simply requiring the objective, experienced and informed gaze of the good nurse, doctor, and social worker, the multidisciplinary team favoured by geriatricians and others concerned with the health and welfare of older people, I have taken a different perspective. Along with other sociological and anthropological studies of medical practices (cf. Becker & Kaufman 1995, Berg 1992, Buckholdt & Gubrium 1979, Silverman 1987) the position taken is that there is far more at stake to how health professionals make their distinctions and categorise people as patients for treatment and care. Further, in my approach, while following in the interpretative tradition, I also seek to press understanding, to explain conduct. By considering how professionals (and patients) are members of societies, organisations and institutions, I examine their practices as cultural performances, through which their identity as members (of disciplines, professions, institutions) or as patients, is not finally ever only conferred, but continuously produced.

Jane Robinson

Professor Celia Davies, occupational sociologist, nurse historian, and friend, on the occasion of my retirement in August 1997 (exactly

45 years after starting work as a student orthopaedic nurse 3 months before my 17th birthday) described my age group of nurses as coming from a 'middle generation'. Before us, she said, were a group of women (for they were almost all women) who not only 'cared for the sick as nurses, but devised arrangements for the running of hospitals and set up district nursing associations. They lived for their work and their dedication and commitment were manifest to all who worked alongside them. Their practical sense and experience triumphed over an impoverished education.' Behind them, Celia observed, 'came a generation for whom educational opportunities were greater. Nursing lost some who might earlier have chosen this field. But nursing kept many whose families felt it improper that women should aspire to medicine or the sciences, or chose to invest their limited resources in educating sons rather than daughters. A nurse training gave board and lodging and commitment laced with pragmatism brought many women of keen intelligence and leadership capacity into nursing.'

It is this 'middle' generation with which I identify. In 1952, when I entered nursing, even the first degree programme in nursing at Edinburgh was still more than a decade away. The second, at Manchester, was almost 20 years from its future foundation. On entering nursing I was immediately aware of what I had given up by (what appeared then) abandoning any chance of entering higher education. Despite the genuine sense of personal satisfaction which I derived from being competent to deliver good nursing care, nothing could make up for the lack of intellectual stimulation. In my case, the decision to abandon the possibility of university education as a consequence of bereavement and subsequent family disinterest was very keenly felt. I 'fell' into nursing as an escape from a personal situation, and I regretted bitterly that having left school before taking 'A' levels, there appeared, for many years, to be no chance of rectifying the situation. Nevertheless, I found the company of my peers congenial, the intellectual demands of nursing relatively easy (I collected several prizes and a gold medal) and, above all, I discovered (to my surprise) that I really enjoyed, and was good at, working with the patients.

I am convinced, however, that the ambivalence which I felt over this early experience turned me into a 'natural' observer. I felt a certain sense of detachment from the professional nursing project and never wanted to be so closely identified with it that I ceased to be my 'own person'. Many years later, Phil Strong, remarkable sociologist, humorist and keen observer of social affairs, commented that natural ethnographers are born, not made, and that they never ever fully 'belong', always remaining on the periphery of the group. I felt that summed up my situation perfectly.

A few salient later experiences feature strongly in my memory. A break from nursing 2 years after registration and following marriage, led to a number of practical opportunities which taught me at first hand about inequalities in health, and social status. Living in Cyprus between 1959 and 1962 in a local community, as an 'RAF (Royal Air Force) wife', I observed the grief and resigned helplessness of women living in extreme poverty when their infants died following episodes of infectious disease, lack of professional help with child bearing, and indifferent or totally absent medical care. As a result, I did not believe then, or now, that however one may occasionally resent their professional attitudes, effective doctors will ever be dispensable.

The practical sociology which I learned as a result of this experience can be summed up in an example of the British class system which led to service wives' medical notes and hospital bed label in the Army Medical Service to read 'wife of Sergeant (Private, Corporal, etc.) Robinson'. To be identified only by one's husband's social status and treated accordingly was a truly educational experience. It was in particular the combination of these two observed situations: the complex interaction of poverty with disease and premature death; and the construction by health professionals of the moral character of their patients by observations on their social status, which led me to appreciate how some patients in receipt of medical and nursing care are judged to be less deserving than others. This had two effects on my subsequent nursing practice. First, I was extremely angry on behalf of patients (especially women) when I felt that their personal integrity was diminished by the forms of medical or nursing care which they received. Second, I became a fierce defender of their right both to be heard and treated appropriately.

The lessons from those experiences have never left me. They were to provide a powerful framework of understanding when I came to research how recipients of health care view the service which they receive, and to realise that the 'inverse care law' (Hart 1971) continues to operate through systems of implicit, socially constructed prejudice. The experiences provided a powerful backdrop to my later studies and also made me aware of the ethical responsibility which one assumes when undertaking research. When identifying uncomfortable research results which suggest that the health services provided are not quite of the order that the health professionals claim, or that their justifications for relatively poor results may be viewed from an alternative perspective, then the researcher has a higher duty to the observed 'truth' than to the personal sensitivities of the professionals (Robinson 1994). Although I have always tried to unravel the underlying explanations for relative variations in observed performance, my personal stance on this particular matter has on occasions, perhaps understandably, resulted in resentment by my fellow health professionals. I see this issue as a major unresolved matter for many nurse researchers who sometimes appear to underestimate the minefield which they enter when undertaking studies of health services in what they believe to be the disinterested pursuit of truth.

Later, when following the health visitors' course in 1969/70 at the University of Keele, my eyes were opened to the possible theoretical interpretations of my personal experiences. The eclectic (and often changing) theoretical underpinnings of contemporary health care practice which I began to learn about then, seemed to me to resemble a complex patchwork quilt which is being constantly re-stitched and added to by contributions from academic disciplines ranging from the biological sciences, epidemiology, statistics, psychology, sociology and social policy. Hence, I became a committed multidisciplinarian. I was convinced that because it is impossible in any one lifetime for a single individual to comprehend the subtleties of all the disciplines involved, it is essential to find common means of discourse between them so that all involved can make their contribution to unravelling and explaining the underlying issues of health and health care. I think that this pragmatic standpoint has much in common with Mark's idea (discussed above) that our shared intellectual tradition allows us enough resources to engage in a dialogue about the kind of society we live in, and the kind of society we ought to have. This is the *complementary interpretations* referred to in the subtitle of this book.

The experience of the health visitor course also crystallised for me the longing which I had for intellectual frameworks for my practice. The course encouraged lateral and critical thinking and, through skilful methods of assessment, encouraged students to explore and expand their knowledge. This was, for me, a major turning point.

Really listening and 'hearing' the 'stories' of those with whom one practices or researches, and identifying the structural forces which shape their interpretations of 'reality' was to become a fundamental tenet of my research. Later, when Head of Department at the University of Nottingham, it also gave me a sense of privilege to work with people such as the co-authors of *Interdisciplinary Perspectives on Health Policy and Practice: competing interests or complementary interpretations?* who were, in their research, extending the necessary theory and the methods much further than I had done. This experience of encouraging others' intellectual development has always been a most valuable part of the rich intrinsic reward one gains from working with colleagues and students in higher education.

As a result of the stimulation derived from the health visitor course, I was to enjoy for 12 of the next 15 years between 1970 and 1985 an experience which will be familiar for many nurses; being a part-time student in higher education with a full-time job, a husband, and a growing family. At the end of this period I had completed two pieces of critical social policy research into aspects of health care practice which earned me a Master's degree and a PhD, and I had embarked upon a third, as director of the Nursing Policy Studies Centre at the University of Warwick. The educational experiences had changed me completely as a person, and as a health care professional, and left me feeling wiser but sadder. If delivery of the best possible health care is so tightly bound up with combating inherent social prejudice, combined with a fear, or inability, seriously to address the foundations of inequalities in health, it appears that all the research in the world on evidence-based practice is unlikely to change the fundamental, hierarchical, nature of health care systems. A large part of the solution must lie therefore in developing the essential catalyst of appropriately educated, visionary and committed health care personnel who will not hold back from confronting the reality, 'warts and all', of their practice.

The eclectic theoretical origins of critical social policy have therefore always provided me with frameworks for research, and also for deriving comfort from their explanations when changing the world has not appeared to be a viable option! For example, when trying first to comprehend and then to offer explanations for the chequered history of health visiting from the end of the 19th century until 1980, identifying a framework which did not just accept that a policy issue become a 'problem' by some invisible process, but instead was the subject of various political strategies (the issue's legitimation, its apparent feasibility, and the level of support) was to provide a model for policy analysis across a range of subjects (Hall et al 1978, Robinson 1982). These approaches to health policy are reflected in the subject matter of my chapters (1 and 2).

Michael Traynor

In January 1991, I started work at the Royal College of Nursing on a 4-year research project aimed at examining the impact of the reforms that were to be unleashed upon the National Health Service in April of that year. The research attempted to measure the job satisfaction of the nursing workforce in four of the first wave of NHS community-based trusts and, alongside this, to produce descriptions of what we spoke of as 'managerial strategy' in the same organisations. The methods involved questionnaire administration (with a form subsequently known, rather imperiously, as The Measure of Job Satisfaction), data gathering at staff meetings and a series of interviews with managers. Repeated at yearly intervals, the intention was to monitor what we imagined would be four crucial, and probably turbulent, years for nursing and the NHS. It seemed likely that the reforms would feature an intensification of the competing interests between the traditional professions and a rising managerialism that the Griffiths reforms of nearly 10 years before had brought to a sharp focus.

My own interests and background eventually led me to concentrate less on numerical comparisons of job satisfaction and more on the written comments nurses added to our questionnaire, the field notes of nursing meetings and, most interestingly perhaps, the transcripts of the 51 interviews I had with trust managers. These sources of data revealed in glorious and grim detail the local operation of a sometimes strident managerialist project and the often outraged, perhaps even rearguard, response of nurses involved in care delivery. At a loss for an analytical or theoretical approach with which to come at these texts, I found myself drawing on the techniques that I had used as a student of literature to open up a Donne sonnet, for example, and make visible the subtle mechanisms of its power and persuasiveness. I will argue later for the value of looking at what might be considered the spontaneous utterances of health service employees in a similar way to the carefully crafted lines of the poet.

At the same time, troubled by issues involving research knowledge, I was reading philosophers like Richard Rorty and Michel Foucault who can be considered central figures in postmodern or poststructuralist thought, from Anglo-American and Continental perspectives respectively. They were trying to tease our picture of knowledge away from any foundation that might be seen as standing outside history and culture and reveal it as contingent as well as implicated in, and giving rise to, various structures of power. Whatever else was going on in the four trusts under study, strongly competing knowledge claims were being made by managers and nursing staff. These claims appeared central to their promotion of their own interests. Postmodern philosophy offered accounts of knowledge which put this struggle into a startling historical and philosophical context, one which I will explain in my chapters (5 and 6).

Unsurprisingly, this kind of reading led me into a deep scepticism about all claims to knowledge, including those made by researchers. Like those literary theorists influenced by a tendency that became known as deconstruction, who make no differentiation between the status of the literary text under study and the critic's own commentary, I claim no detached position from which to represent the texts of managers and nurses. What I do claim, as do all the collaborators in this book, is a rigour that is immanent to the different fields of practice in which we work.

One approach to research that focuses on the activity of language itself has become known as discourse analysis. Approaches such as discourse analysis change the focus of inquiry from the individual and his or her thoughts and intention to language itself which makes available the very categories of thought and representation. The speech of the managers and nurses cannot be explained simply by notions of individual intention.

In other words we can approach the texts not as the more or less neutral channel of communication from the consciousness of an individual who utters them out into the world, but as embodiments of discourses that in a sense pre-exist and are *participated in* by individuals and institutions as part of the not necessarily conscious advancement of their interests. Discourses provide positions that can be adopted, spaces that can be occupied, categories that can be available as well as those which are prohibited. For example, the language and very notion of 'self-sacrifice' provides a powerful position available for nurses as they seek to represent themselves in a way that counter-balances (what they see as) the rhetoric of managers. For the managers, their self-characterisation as bringers of rationality to a realm of traditional practice depends, in part, for its power upon already existing discourses. I would argue that, in a sense, discourse comes before individuality because there is no way of getting at human subjectivity or no way to approach self-understanding that can side-step discourse, available ways of thinking about and speaking about ourselves. This is why both groups, again, not necessarily con-sciously, sought to identify their interests with some foundational discourse.

Of course, one of the major contexts of this research is political; both the champions of the reforms who took up the challenge to lead their organisations into a new future and those nurses in the same organisations who were sceptical, for a whole range of reasons, had much at stake, more than just their personal satisfaction. The managers had become major stakeholders in the Government's reforms while many of the nurses, in their own argumentation, echoed the language and discursive strategies used by the Royal College of Nursing a decade before in its high-profile, and high-cost, campaign against the Griffiths reorganisation.

The reader may now be experiencing a sense of irritation at my dichotomous use of the terms 'nurse' and 'manager'. What about the role of the trust nurse executive, promoted by the NHS Executive itself as a potentially powerful figure representing nursing at trust board level (NHSME 1992)? What about the many nurses in middle management positions? Regarding the latter, whose position I will not be examining in any depth in these chapters, I suggest that their predicament was the most pressured, placed between the expecta-tions, often of a financial nature, from above yet still exposed, if not to the experience of care delivery, to the stress and distress of 'front-line' nurses who were. Regarding the nurse executives, I will argue, using the interview material as my evidence, that while they attempted to combine nursing and managerialist discourses, their argumenta-tion aligned far more with a managerialist orientation than it did with the positions taken by front-line nurses or nursing's professional organisations.

CONCLUSION

With these biographical details of the four authors in place, each now contributes two chapters to *Interdisciplinary Perspectives on Health Policy and Practice: competing interests or complementary interpretations?* written from the perspectives which they have outlined. The final chapter will pull together the ideas and discuss the lessons which may be learned from a project of this nature.

REFERENCES

Barnes B, Edge D 1982 Science in context: readings in the sociology of science. Open University Press, Milton Keynes
Baruch G 1981 Moral tales: parents stories of encounters with the health profession. Sociology of Health and Illness 3(3): 275–296
Becker G, Kaufman S R 1995 Managing an uncertain illness trajectory in old age: patients' and physicians' views of stroke. Medical Anthropology Quarterly 9(2): 165–187
Berg M 1992 The construction of medical disposals. Medical sociology and medical problem-solving in clinical practice. Sociology of Health and Illness 14(2): 151–180
Buckholdt D R, Gubrium J F 1979 Doing staffings. Human Organisation 38(3): 255–264
Clay T 1987 Nurses: power and politics. Heinemann, London
Davidson D 1984 Inquiries into truth and interpretation. Oxford University Press, Oxford
Davies C 1980 A constant casualty: nurse education in Britain and the USA to 1939. In: Davies C (ed) Rewriting nursing history. Croom Helm, London
Descartes R 1637 Discourse on method and The meditations. Penguin Books, London, 1968
Fairclough N 1992 Discourse and text: linguistic and intertextual analysis within discourse analysis. Discourse and Society 3(2): 193–217
Fairclough N 1993 Critical discourse analysis and the marketization of public discourse. Discourse and Society 4(2): 133–168
Fernandez J W 1986a Persuasions and performances: of the beast in every body and the metaphors of every man. In: Fernandez J W Persuasions and performances: the play of tropes in culture. Indiana University Press, Bloomington
Fernandez J W 1986b Introduction. In: Fernandez J W Persuasions and performances: the play of tropes in culture. Indiana University Press, Bloomington
Goodman N 1983 Fact, fiction, and forecast. MIT Press, Cambridge Mass
Hall P, Land H, Parker R, Webb A 1978 Change, choice and conflict in social policy. Heinemann, London
Hardy L K 1986 Career politics: the case of career histories of selected leading female and male nurses in England and Scotland. In: White R (ed) Political issues in nursing: past, present and future. Wiley, Chichester, vol 2, ch 4, pp 69–82
Hart J T 1971 The inverse care law. Lancet i: 405–412
Kuhn T 1970 The structure of scientific revolutions. University of Chicago Press, Chicago
Latimer J 1998a Organising context: nurses' assessments of older people in an acute medical unit. Nursing Inquiry 5(1): 43–57
Latimer J 1998b The dark at the bottom of the stair: participation and performance of older people in hospital. Medical Anthropology Quarterly (in press)
Locke J 1964 An essay concerning human understanding. Fontana, London
Luntley M 1995 Reason, truth and self: the postmodern reconditioned. Routledge, London

Lyotard J F 1985 The postmodern condition: a report on knowledge. Manchester University Press, Manchester

Marcus G, Fischer M 1986 Anthropology as cultural critique: an experimental moment in the human sciences. Chicago University Press, Chicago

National Health Service Management Executive (NHSME) 1992 One year on: the nurse executive director post. Report on the role and function of the nurse executive director post in first wave NHS trusts. Department of Health and the Central Office of Information, London

Paley J 1997 Husserl, phenomenology and nursing. Journal of Advanced Nursing 26: 187–193

Putnam H 1981 Reason, truth and history. Cambridge University Press, Cambridge

Quine W 1960 Word and object. MIT Press, Cambridge Mass

Quine W V O 1980 From a logical point of view. Harvard University Press, Cambridge Mass

Rafferty A-M 1996 The politics of nursing knowledge. Routledge, London

Robinson J 1982 An evaluation of health visiting. Council for the Education and Training of Health Visitors/English National Board for Nursing, Midwifery and Health Visiting, London

Robinson J 1991 Power, politics and policy analysis in nursing. In: Perry A, Jolley M (eds) Nursing: a knowledge base for practice. Edward Arnold, London, ch 9, pp 271–307

Robinson J 1994 Research for whom? The politics of research dissemination and application. In: Buckledee J, McMahon R (eds) The research experience in nursing. Chapman and Hall, London, ch 11, pp 165–188

Robinson J, Gray A, Elkan R (eds) 1992 Policy issues in nursing. Open University Press, Milton Keynes

Rorty R 1991 Objectivity, relativism, and truth. Cambridge University Press, Cambridge

Royal College of Nursing (RCN) 1997 Congress 1997: Agenda Item 15: That this meeting of the RCN congress supports the introduction of political education as an integral part of pre-registration courses (submitted by the RCN Association of Nursing Students). RCN, London

Said E W 1994 Representations of the intellectual. Pantheon, New York

Salvage J 1985 The politics of nursing. Heinemann, London

Silverman D 1987 Communication and medical practice. Social relations in the clinic. Sage, London

Silverman D 1993 Interpreting qualitative data. Methods for analysing talk, text and interaction. Sage, London

Silverman D 1997 Discourses of counselling. HIV counselling as social interaction. Sage, London

Simnett A 1986 The pursuit of respectability: women and the nursing profession, 1860–1900. In: White R (ed) Political issues in nursing: past, present and future. Wiley, Chichester, vol 2, ch 1, pp 1–17

Strathern M 1991 Partial connections. Rowman and Littlefield, Savage Md

Strathern M 1992 After nature. English kinship in the late twentieth century. Cambridge University Press, Cambridge

Strathern M 1994 Pre-figured features: A view from the Papua New Guinea Highlands. In: Woodall J (ed) The visual construction of identity. Manchester University Press, Manchester

Strathern M 1995 The relation. Issues in complexity and scale. Prickly Pear Press, Cambridge

Strong P, Robinson J 1990 The NHS under new management. Open University Press, Milton Keynes

Turner V 1967 The forest of symbols: aspects of Ndembu ritual. Cornell University Press, Ithaca NY

Tyler S A 1986 Post-modern ethnography: from document of the occult to occult document. In: Clifford J, Marcus G (eds) Writing culture: the poetics and politics of ethnography. California University Press, Berkeley, Los Angeles

Van Fraassen B 1980 The scientific image. Oxford University Press, Oxford

White R (ed) 1985 Political issues in nursing: past, present and future. Wiley, Chichester, vol 1

White R (ed) 1986 Political issues in nursing: past, present and future. Wiley, Chichester, vol 2

White R (ed) 1988 Political issues in nursing: past, present and future. Wiley, Chichester, vol 3

Winch P 1958 The idea of a social science. Routledge and Kegan Paul, London

Wittgenstein L 1953 Philosophical investigations. Basil Blackwell, Oxford

Researching National Health Service reform in the 1980s: issues of substance and method

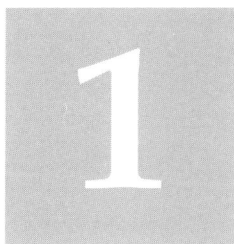

Jane Robinson

■ **CONTENTS**

Introduction 33
The research context 34
The NHS: a state of continuous reform? 35
The Griffiths' reforms and the introduction of general management to the NHS 37

Making sense of our data 41
Explaining the situation 43
The national survey of Chief Nurse Advisors 45
Conclusion 47
References 50

INTRODUCTION

This chapter draws on the experience of a 3-year study carried out between 1985 and 1988 under the auspices of the Nursing Policy Studies Centre at the University of Warwick, into the management of nursing following the implementation of the Griffiths Inquiry Report into the management of the National Health Service (DHSS 1983, 1984). The Griffiths research (by which shorthand term it became known) was carried out by myself and Philip Strong, an erudite and sophisticated sociologist and ethnographer (Robinson & Strong 1987, Strong & Robinson 1988, 1990). Ruth Elkan contributed to the final report after Phil Strong had left the project (Robinson et al 1989).

This chapter uses aspects of the published research findings together with reflections on the experience of *carrying out* the Griffiths research to consider, with all the benefits of hindsight, the competing interests which can be identified from these examples of National Health Service (NHS) reforms, and on the interpretations which can be made of these interests by researchers from very different backgrounds. I will argue that despite my being the project leader for this research the real, albeit hidden, power relationships between my co-researcher and myself resulted in an interpretation of the research findings which served a dominant view of interests in the NHS. As such, the chapter provides a useful case study on an attempt in the mid-1980s to establish a critical approach to the study of nursing policy. It shows how, in the absence of any developed tradition or resource base in the area, one was very dependent on available expertise which ultimately was shown to have shaped the direction and the interpretation of the findings. The chapter also provides evidence on how a changed organisational framework within the NHS, with an overriding emphasis on *efficiency*, provided the context for the 're-identification' of medical and nursing practice described in Joanna Latimer's and Michael Traynor's chapters. Yet the Griffiths research which is reported in this chapter was not concerned at all with researching clinical practice, it was a study of NHS organisational change and the impact which this had on some of the key players within that organisation.

THE RESEARCH CONTEXT

In January 1985 a small research centre, independently funded by the King Edward VII Hospital Fund for London, was opened in the School of Social Studies at the University of Warwick. Titled the Nursing Policy Studies Centre (NPSC) it had a constitution with three major objectives:

1. To develop the theoretical evaluation of nursing policy
2. To influence the making of policy so that nurses could make the optimal contribution to health service and health care policy in all sectors and at all levels of the health care system
3. To involve nurses and to create greater awareness amongst nurses and others of nursing policy issues (NPSC 1988).

The way in which this task was undertaken is described in Robinson et al (1992). The crucial elements for the purposes of this chapter were first, that despite the Centre's limited, short-term, funding (£164 000 for 4 years' activity) there was provision to make an independent choice of a research topic within the level of this resource. Second, the decision to undertake research into the management of nursing following the Griffiths' reforms of the NHS (DHSS 1983, 1984) was based on a number of expediencies:

- The topic was identified as providing a valuable opportunity to demonstrate to nurses, and others, of what a critical approach to nursing policy might consist.
- The topic, of its nature, demanded the collaborative skills of a social scientist (there was finance for only one additional researcher, and for 3 of the 4 years) who would be able to set the nursing issues within a much wider policy and theoretical context.
- The topic was of relevance to all clinical specialisms in nursing and could not therefore be seen to be showing a preference for any one, for example hospital over community-based nursing.

Third, recruiting a researcher with the appropriate social science skills was a difficult process and almost half of the first precious year had passed before we were able to make an appointment. Phil Strong who took up the post in May 1985 had a reputation as a formidable sociologist who also wrote in language accessible to the non-academic. I could not believe our good fortune in being able to recruit such an expert who was also immensely humorous and like-able. Unsurprisingly, he was 'head-hunted' from elsewhere just before his 3-year contract expired. Despite his relatively short time with the NPSC, Phil Strong was, nevertheless, responsible for many powerful influences on the direction which the Griffiths research took, in partic-ular in seeing health care reform as a part of an immensely long histor-ical process in the development of management in the NHS.

A different perspective on the explanations for such reforms will be developed in Chapter 2 which examines the international trends in ideas which underpin health care reform. What the reflection in this chapter demonstrates is that researching with colleagues with very different theoretical and practical interests can challenge nurses both on their interpretations of research findings, and on the stand which they may be prepared to take on them. The chapter also draws briefly on the experience of earlier research into the evaluation of health visiting which was instigated as the subject of my Master's degree following the NHS Reorganisation Act 1973 (DHSS 1972, Robinson 1982).

THE NHS: A STATE OF CONTINUOUS REFORM?

The term 'NHS reform' tends to be taken as meaning whichever latest reform is currently being discussed. The Labour Government's reforms following the White Papers *The New NHS: modern, dependable* (DoH 1997) and *Our Healthier Nation* (DoH 1998) will no doubt come in time to be referred to in much the same way. However, some accounts see some reforms as much more important than others. For example, Charles Webster, official historian of the NHS, refers to the 1989 White Paper *Working for Patients* (DoH 1989a) as marking 'a fundamental turning point in British health care' (Webster 1993) and describes earlier attempts to reform the NHS as either relatively minor, or (as in the case of the 1974 reforms) 'a failure' (p. 18). Yet, the question arises – important to *whom*? The reforms of 1974 (DHSS 1972), 1982 (DHSS and Welsh Office 1979, DHSS 1980) and 1983 (DHSS 1983, 1984) were all deeply felt by those in practice at the time, certainly by nurses, to be both professionally challenging and, for some, profoundly disruptive to the task of routinely delivering health care.

The 1974 reforms may be seen by some from the viewpoint of history as 'a failure', but for district nurses, health visitors and community midwives, the changes from local authority to NHS control which were implemented then, and which had such a profound effect on subsequent patterns of practice, have never been reversed. For this group of community nurses, whose professional practice had been developed historically as 'autonomous' (albeit with ultimate accountability to, and under the medical control of, the Medical Officer of Health), the 1974 reforms were to bring increasing identification with the caseloads of general medical practice, and managerial subordination to a hospital-dominated NHS.

This particular episode in community nursing history may be seen in the light of subsequent events to have been a model for all the later subtle re-constructions of 'interests' which Joanna Latimer describes in such detail. In creating a vast, inappropriate and expensive management bureaucracy in the NHS, the 1974 reforms may have been a *managerial* failure but they were successful in beginning to 'bring into line' those nurses who had a professional tendency to be independent in thought and action. Michael Traynor's detailed analysis of community nurses' and managers' discourses following the implementation of *Working for Patients* (DoH 1989a) and *Caring for People: community care in the next decade and beyond* (DoH 1989b) demonstrates that the underlying issues still rumble on. It appears then that despite the verdict of history, reforms do ultimately bring about changes, some of which such as *Working for Patients*, have perhaps more visible or profound effects on the overall *management* of the service whilst others have equally profound effects on the behaviour and practices of health professionals. The verdict of history may well see the Griffiths (1983) reforms as having this latter effect on nurse managers.

Such competing views on the practical significance of reform leads one to suspect that anyone who is not personally involved in the daily delivery of services is unlikely to have any notion of the often massive destabilising effect on those in practice of successive changes in philosophy, overall structure, management hierarchies, individual personnel, and financial arrangements. The term 'reform weariness' as a form of post-traumatic stress syndrome has been coined to describe the feelings of staff faced with yet another NHS reform.

So what lies behind the apparent phenomenon of 'constant NHS reform'? The question will be addressed by reflecting on what later transpired to be the often competing perspectives held by Phil Strong and myself on the subject matter of our research. Having experienced working in the NHS during the 1974 and 1982 reforms I came to the reporting of our research findings with the idea that we had to make explicit the often highly traumatised accounts that we were given; Phil Strong, however, held a very different view. He saw reform as providing much needed radical change, and the particular wave of reform which we were observing as an inevitable consequence of needing to improve dramatically on what had gone before. Indeed, as we shall see, he believed that radical reform of the NHS was long overdue.

THE GRIFFITHS' REFORMS AND
THE INTRODUCTION OF
GENERAL MANAGEMENT TO THE NHS

The 1983 NHS reforms were fundamentally about the search for 'value for money' or efficiency. The term 'NHS plc' was widely used amongst senior managers at their conferences early in the implementation process to indicate the business-like character of the new NHS, but Phil Strong set this new ethos within the wider context of the then Conservative Government's philosophy. He noted a speech by

Clive Priestley (a central figure in Mrs Thatcher's attempts to improve the efficiency of the civil service) to the Adam Smith Institute which included the following statement:

> The theory of the welfare state ... has not ... until recently included any emphasis at all on efficiency, effectiveness or value for money. This is a very curious omission, and the fact that it exists is a comment on the relatively slack intellectual times in which we live, as compared with, say, political philosophy one hundred years ago.
>
> (Priestley 1986, pp. 124–125)

Thus efficiency in the NHS became just one strand of the driving government philosophy of the time which returned to 'Victorian values' and discounted the work of the past 30–40 years in terms of the establishment and continuation of the service, and its contribution to the health of the British public.

But, for many health professionals, when the Griffiths reforms were first introduced they were characterised as a perceived attack on the notion of 'consensus management' by a group of 'equals' in the NHS – a manager, a finance officer, a doctor and a nurse, which had been introduced in 1974 (DHSS 1972). This form of senior management was seen by the Griffiths Report to be grossly inefficient because, it was claimed, no-one would ever take the responsibility for making a decision, and ultimately everyone deferred to the doctor. Thus, crucial decisions which needed an immediate response, and longer-term strategic planning, became impossible to make because of the power politics which operated within the 'consensus' group. Roy Griffiths' famous comment in his Report that 'if Florence Nightingale were to be walking the hospitals today she would ask "who is in charge?"' summed up the rationale for the appointment of one 'supremo' – the general manager – in each unit of NHS management.

Line management of health care professionals by senior nurses and members of the professions ancillary to medicine (PAMs) also succumbed to the overall authority of the general managers (some of whom might indeed be 'former' nurses or PAMs). Medicine itself had never been subject to line management, but the introduction of general management implied that doctors too would be expected after 1983 to be subject to the overall *managerial* decisions of the general manager. Later experience was to prove that the dividing line between managerial and clinical decisions was a fine one indeed for many doctors. Medical recalcitrance had to be dealt with (we later concluded that Griffiths had actually been conceived as an attack upon the doctors but that 'nursing was caught in the crossfire'). Hence, the notion of 'clinical management' was heavily endorsed in later developments, epitomised by the replacement of the term 'management budgeting' by 'clinical budgeting'. By such processes, medical clinicians were recruited to subscribe to the new discourses of efficiency and financial management. Their interests were realigned and their identities managed. How these discourses were then played out later in clinical practice with both the development of competing discourses and the modification of professional behaviours, is described in their respective chapters (5–8) by Michael Traynor and Joanna Latimer.

The loss of senior line management posts previously held by nurses gave rise to much outcry in the nursing press. The purchase by the Royal College of Nursing (RCN) of a full page spread in the Sunday Times to ask whether 'the general manager knows his coccyx from his humerus?' may have put the RCN in a new light in terms of its ability to use the media, but the campaign proved to be almost completely unsuccessful in stemming the tide of change (Robinson 1992, p. 1). The reasons for nursing's dissatisfaction with the introduction of general management had several strands. First, it was argued that for most of the time nurses *were* the managers of continuous clinical processes in the NHS. Nurses, it was claimed, know the warp and the weft of health care, they are 'in touch' with all the realities of health care practice, therefore they should be recognised for the managerial role which they undoubtedly play. Joanna Latimer in Chapter 8 maintains that this remains the case, with nurses discretely 'managing' on-call situations, throughput and 'bed-blockers'. Second, junior nurses needed the professional support and guidance of more senior colleagues – how could anyone who was *not* a nurse possibly understand about nursing matters, let alone give professional advice? Third, there was the issue of the loss of a managerial career structure and potential future opportunities for nurses. (This issue tended to be dealt with by managers by pointing out the huge opportunities in general management which existed for those with the potential to convert to the new ways of thinking.) Finally, and crucially, senior nurses felt a profound sense of injustice when relegated to a purely advisory role, having previously managed comparatively vast budgets for the nursing services. Others, it has to be said, appeared to rise to the new situation, stating that they saw it as a considerable, positive, challenge for nursing, and one of our research tasks was to try to identify the reasons for these different attitudes and forms of behaviour.

The question of the budget lay, however, at the heart of many of our early interviews with senior nurses. To some, the loss of financial control represented the total loss of power which was expressed by some nurses as a sense of bereavement during our first round of interviews. 'Money *is* power' was a view expressed to us with some vehemence by one respondent in the study. This was not seen just as a loss of *personal* power but also as a genuine *fear* that once the financial purse strings for the nursing workforce were held by someone who neither knew nor cared about nursing, then the consequence would be the demise of any further development of the profession. (At the time of the research, Chief Nursing Officers at District Health Authority (DHA) level also held the nurse education budget, a resource which was to revert to the Regional Health Authorities, and then to educational commissioning consortia, several years later.) Respondents reported that it was widely rumoured that during the planning of the implementation of general management, one senior government official had said, 'Oh yes, the nursing budget, that is the *real* prize!'

It has to be remembered that this official's reported statement was absolutely true. In representing 50% of the workforce and approximately 30% of the budget, nursing expenditure ran into many millions of pounds in every DHA. Nurses were frequently in control of the largest single budget and the Griffiths' reforms were above all about the search for 'value for money' or efficiency. It was, therefore, hardly surprising that control of such a large resource was wrested from the nurses and placed with general management as a consequence of the 1983 Griffiths reforms.

The response of many of the senior nurses who felt so cheated by what had happened to them in the Griffiths reorganisation was that these things could not be allowed to happen as there were *statutory* responsibilities which had to be met by senior nurse managers. Phil Strong saw this as an unsubstantiated ploy; not so much a moral argument as a 'red herring' introduced by nurses in defence of their interests, and he quickly disposed of it in our first report (Robinson & Strong 1987).

A related feature of the 1983 reforms involved the need to institute appropriate information systems so that all the elements of the service could be centrally monitored. As the Managing Director for Sainsbury Supermarkets, Roy Griffiths was reported to be appalled to discover that it was virtually impossible to identify the unit cost of any item of service in the NHS. Thus, the gauntlet thrown to health professionals was the challenge to identify the most cost-effective ways of delivering their services, and this situation led to an explosion of interest in the various ways of monitoring nursing quality against cost. The economics of nursing was at a primitive stage of development and, understandably, both nurses and the new general managers looked to the only country in the world which had pioneered the development of such monitoring systems, the United States of America (USA). The fact that many of these systems had been instituted in order to facilitate the billing process in a health system with a large private health care sector, only added to the worries of many professionals that what the NHS had traditionally 'stood for' as a service free at the point of delivery was now under sustained attack.

MAKING SENSE OF OUR DATA

Phil Strong brought to our research a formidable grasp of the enormously long sweeps of history in which he believed it is essential to contextualise the political occurrences of today. He spent many hours talking to a political philosopher on the significance of what we were observing, and when the final account of our research came to be written as *The NHS Under New Management* he began the Foreword with the following statement:

> Between 1837 and 1841, so it appears, George Whistler introduced the first modern management system into business …. Whistler was the Superintendent of the Western Railroad of Boston, Massachusetts …. He placed himself and a small headquarters staff at the hub of the organization. The rest he separated into three operating divisions: engineering, transport and maintenance. The new principle he introduced to the business was that of continuous accountability: detailed management was delegated to the divisions but it was simultaneously made subject to constant, systematic monitoring. Each division had to report on a daily, weekly and monthly basis, supplying financial and performance data to the central office staff for their regular appraisal and (where necessary) intervention.
>
> (Strong & Robinson 1990, p. ix)

Thus Phil Strong saw the introduction of general management into the NHS as a part of an inevitable and long overdue social process which had originated early in the 19th century in the teaching of assessment and management at West Point Military Academy, USA (where Whistler was a cadet). The only surprise was that it had taken so long before such managerial methods had crossed the divide from the commercial to the public sector.

When we were preparing the first report following the piloting phase of the research (Robinson & Strong 1987) I expressed concern that it would be unethical not to include reference to the distress which we had observed amongst some senior nurses. Phil Strong was unequivocally opposed. The only thing, he said, which mattered was improving the quality of NHS performance. If nurses had not 'come up to scratch' in developing and monitoring quality standards in nursing, then they were inevitable victims in the onward march of progress. Thus, our only reference to the consequences to nurse managers of the introduction of such radical and rapid change was the following statement on two immediate costs to nursing:

> First, there is the loss of experienced senior talent. No doubt some of those who have gone had serious flaws: this much seems fairly common ground. But every reshuffle allows the winners to settle old scores, sometimes unjustly – the good often go with the bad. Second, nursing has lost some of its hard won autonomy. The independent control of its own affairs has long been one of the profession's central goals in its search for professional status ... But if its partial loss now matters to nurses, does it matter at all to patients?
>
> (Robinson & Strong 1987, p. vi)

At the time, there appeared to be an irrefutable logic in such statements. Nursing clearly needed a revolution in terms of providing the evidence for its cost-effectiveness. Within just over 1 year from the inception of the study and at the end of our piloting phase, the overall conceptual framework for our research was thus determined; the study had to be predominantly about improving quality and developing standards in the NHS. For nursing, this had to be addressed in terms of what was known, and should be known, about nursing's effectiveness and efficiency. As far as nurse managers were concerned, if they were not producing the evidence on these issues, then they had no claim to be managers anyway. Phil Strong was not unsympathetic to the nurses' situation; indeed he believed that nurses should be given far more authority and responsibility for the management and delivery of health care. To achieve this, however, he also believed that nurses should take on the reality and the relevance of the new situation and develop nursing accordingly to conform to the demands of the new era. This meant developing its knowledge base and becoming more businesslike in its approach to value for money in the delivery of a nursing service.

EXPLAINING THE SITUATION

The second phase of our study focused on how the need for change in the light of the reforms was being handled. A few remarkable examples were identified where senior nurses were working in very dynamic ways to develop methods of monitoring quality and ensuring that nurses made a significant contribution to clinical developments. We observed that, in general, these 'new wave' nurses were working in authorities which had become government 'flagships' for the new order. The most senior nurses working in these settings had themselves experienced the benefits of higher education, and either they, or their general managers, had instigated a search for some of the most able nurses to work with them in their health authority. Above all, these senior nurses appeared to enjoy considerable informed support both from lay authority board members (including chairpersons) and, perhaps partly as a consequence of this, support from their general managers.

On the whole, however, after 3 years of research, we had to report that once much of the initial excitement over the Griffiths reforms had subsided, most aspects of nursing remained a 'black hole'. The tensions to which this situation gave rise – the nursing group locked into the gravitational force of its internal preoccupations and the others, on the outside, unable or unwilling to look in and comprehend the nature of nursing's dilemmas, seemed to us to be the social equivalent of an astronomical black hole (Robinson 1992, p. 5). Phil Strong was no feminist and virtually his only 'nod' in the direction of gender as an explanation for this phenomenon was that 'Doctors, managers and men have other priorities' (Strong & Robinson 1988, p. 158). We held many inconclusive discussions on the mechanisms which gave rise to this state of affairs. Phil Strong saw the problem simply in terms of a 'water and diamonds' analogy – nursing skills are plentiful, like water; brain surgeons are scarce, like diamonds.

We concluded the second report with an analysis of the current demographic situation which suggested that the numbers of recruits into nursing would continue to fall whilst the demand for nursing services in the light of an ageing population was almost certain to rise. We argued that this potential contraction of the size of the nursing labour force could work to its advantage. Phil Strong observed that 'you can't have a profession with half a million members.' He believed that a smaller group would offer the opportunity for better education; better appropriation of appropriate jobs for nurses; and delegation to the less qualified.

In support of this argument we also drew attention to the powerful historical differences between nursing and medicine and the need, if anything was to change, for nurses to begin to redress the balance. We collected together the 'mirror image' of the stereotypes which characterise both professions:

> Doctors are men and nurses are women; doctors are small in number but possess extraordinary power; nursing is vast in size but amazingly weak in influence; doctors are educated and nurses are ignorant; doctors are wealthy, nurses are poorly paid; doctors have a vast scientific base, nursing has hardly any; doctors are independent professionals, possessing a fierce autonomy of judgement, nursing is not a profession and has been notorious for its hierarchy, indeed almost a military discipline; doctors are famed for their solidarity when threatened, nurses renowned for the ease with which they give way. Viewed together, the two trades have a strange symmetry; each is a bizarre image of the other.
>
> (Strong & Robinson 1988, p. 20)

Davies (1995) later took us to task for not making explicit some of the issues of power and control which our analysis had revealed; that 'in the defensiveness and uncertainty of nurses managers themselves there is a failure to acknowledge that there is a management job to be done' (p. 165). She points out that making a transition to a progressive model is not something which will be achieved merely by exhorting nurses; that it is: 'part and parcel of the dilemma of devaluation of their (nurses') work as 'women's work' – something we are not used to seeing as in need of management. The work that women do, after all, is noticed when it is not there, and taken for granted when it is' (Davies 1995, p. 165).

Celia Davies was quite correct. The competing interests which we had identified between doctors and nurses, and nurses and managers, were based on an analysis which failed to take into account the structural forces, in particular gender, which shape occupations and the value which is placed on them. In struggling to begin to develop a critical approach to the study of nursing policy at Warwick and to recruit intellectual expertise to the project, I had become submerged by the weight of another's *a priori* convictions concerning the nature of the problem in relation only as it applied to general management. Phil Strong's deeply held convictions on the nature of the problem discounted the need to analyse in far greater depth the structural sources of power which were played out between the different groups of workers in the health care system and, in particular, how nurses were subordinated in the process.

THE NATIONAL SURVEY OF
CHIEF NURSE ADVISORS

The conclusions which we drew for the first and second reports were based on data collected between 1985 and 1987 from wide-ranging observations and interviews with some 152 senior NHS employees, government department officials, and health authority members, as well as attendance at 11 conferences on the subject of NHS management. Our major focus had been on seven health authorities in England and Wales selected partly on the basis of their population (and therefore budget) size, and partly on the management arrangements which had been instituted for nursing after the Griffiths Report was implemented. By the late summer of 1987 we had a large volume of data which Phil Strong began systematically to analyse. From this our second report was written (Strong & Robinson 1988). As he had an equally strong interest in the subject of general management *per se* the idea of a book based on the considerable amount of evidence which we held was also proposed. Thus the idea of *The NHS Under New Management* was born (Strong & Robinson 1990).

I was not satisfied, however, that our findings should be based on a relatively small sample of health authorities (however vast the data collection may have appeared to us at the time). I therefore designed a 66-question questionnaire using the ideas generated from our main qualitative study which was distributed to every Chief Nurse Advisor (CNA) in England and Wales. Wales was of particular interest for it was a proud Welsh claim that their chief nurses retained the 'officer' part of their title (Chief Advisory Nursing Officer) as an indication that they had retained greater management control of nursing than was the case for their English counterparts. The survey received a response rate of 81%, being returned by 156 senior nurses from 193 health authorities.

The results of the survey *Griffiths and the Nurses: a national survey of CNAs* (Robinson et al 1989) was published in the Nursing Policy Studies Series as our third 'Griffiths' report. By this time Phil Strong had left to become director of the History of AIDS Research Unit at the London School of Hygiene and Tropical Medicine and I was struggling to maintain the Nursing Policy Studies Centre on 'soft' research monies. The excitement with which we had begun the study of the management of nursing following the implementation of the Griffiths Inquiry Report had been dissipated by the exhaustion which resulted from the scale of the qualitative work undertaken, and the lack of resources to carry on and disseminate further our findings. As a result, the findings from the national survey made nothing like the impact which our earlier reports had done. Yet, *Griffiths and the Nurses* represents an important statement on the degree to which nursing in England and Wales had been seriously disempowered following the introduction of general management. If the original intention of Griffiths had been to control the clinical spending power of the medical profession, it had reached only an uneasy compromise with the doctors. Senior nursing staff on the other hand had been decimated. Of course it was not fashionable, or even wise, to say so. Anyone who hankered after past models of management was seen as out of touch with reality, as old fashioned as the images of nursing they generated, with their connotations of rigid hierarchy and rather foolish women in frilly caps.

In the results of the 1988 survey, carried out 5 years after the Griffiths Report of 1983, we found no common principles or unifying factors underpinning the rationales for the provision of nursing advice to district general managers, or to DHAs. 29 different job titles were reported from the 156 nurses who responded to the question-naire and only 20 (12.6%) retained a post at district level which had no other responsibility apart from nursing. 73 (46.8%) combined the giving of nursing advice with 201 reported general management functions. These included quality assurance, personnel, workforce planning, training and information management. There was little evidence that these nurses had received further education and training for these new responsibilities, although several reported that they had, or were in the process of completing, Master's degrees in Business Administration, Public Policy, and Public Sector Management. 12 (7.5%) CNAs combined their posts with that of the Director of Nurse Education. 63 (42.6%) health authorities had no established nursing support posts at all, 70 (47.3%) had one or two. Not surprisingly, two-thirds of the respondents thought that the situation was worse at the time of replying than before the implementation of Griffiths, and only 5% thought that it was better.

Two-thirds of CNAs reported that not only did they have no access to the informal power structures (the 'kitchen cabinets') in the health authority, but also their access to routine managerial and research-based information was extremely limited. (It will be recalled that prior to the 1983 reforms these senior nurses would have been members of consensus management teams at DHA levels.) More than 50% of respondents reported ward closures because of financial stringency and 48% because of staff shortages. Yet less than half reported having 'great freedom' to develop proactive manpower strategies. Only a quarter of CNAs perceived their professional role to have been strengthened since Griffiths. There was, however, a great diversity of views and many CNAs cited their admiration for their nursing colleagues who had coped magnificently in the face of poor morale and financial difficulties.

CONCLUSION

Does this somewhat depressing evidence on the decline of senior nursing's influence *matter* a decade after it was collected, with a further NHS reorganisation past down the road, and a new one on the horizon? Phil Strong would have said 'only if it matters to patients'. I would suggest, however, that the situation is more complicated than that, for there are demonstrated beneficial connections between nurses' sense of autonomy and control over their work and a wish to stay in an health care organisation, and even on the death rates of patients (Aiken & Sloane 1997, Aiken et al 1994, 1997, American Public Health Association 1997).

There are other reasons too. First, the marginal attention which the third report on the Griffiths research from the Nursing Policy Studies

Centre received at the time it was published was not just a function of an exhausted researcher without the time to disseminate the findings. Readers do not like having to digest bad news and in the political climate prevailing at that time, the findings could easily be attributed to 'special pleading'. The two earlier 'Griffiths' reports were qualitative and 'up beat'; the second full of outrageous, often very funny, quotations with which most readers could identify. Indeed, the humour may possibly have had a beneficial effect on the psychological functioning of some of those traumatised by the very changes we had described, by encouraging people to laugh at themselves. Once a situation has been converted into a funny anecdote, made public, and everyone has had a laugh because they can identify with the nub of the joke, tension is relieved and there is a sense of not being alone any more. However, as the old adage 'many a true word spoken in jest' implies, the joke does not diminish the seriousness of the reality behind the story.

The presentation of the first two 'Griffiths' reports took as their model for reporting the same enthusiastic and somewhat 'zany' approach as those health service managers who had most ardently advocated the Griffiths reforms. But in the face of this cheerful 'style' it was relatively easy not to take the messages about nursing too seriously. In presenting our research in this way we may have contributed to the 'up beat' philosophy which has since been adopted, apparently of necessity, by all those who have climbed the 'slippery pole' to nurse management positions since Griffiths. 'Bad news' is simply not allowed. It is letting the side down. This may be seen to be either British 'stiff upper lip' or a sensible approach to job security. It does nothing to expose the soft underbelly of the current reality of British nursing.

In retrospect, I felt a sense of responsibility for not adhering to Said's (1994) challenge to the intellectual to analyse and take a stronger stand on the position of the minority, the unrepresented and the invisible. The Griffiths research undertaken by Phil Strong and myself may, in some small part, have contributed to the prevailing notion that a cheerful face has to be put on any situation in nursing and health care. This stance may have silenced any hope of critical research which attempts to convey a realistic picture of what is happening in nursing. Soundings made about the possibility of replicating the approach to the Griffiths research following the implementation of *Working for Patients* (DoH 1989) met with no interest whatsoever. Hence, after a brief moment of visibility during the 3 years we were conducting the Griffiths research, nursing, as an *organisational* issue, has been forced back into the shadows. Does this matter to patients? The trouble is we simply do not know. However, if research carried out at the micro level of analysis such as that reported by Joanna Latimer in Chapters 7 and 8 is anything to go by, these organisational issues continue to impinge in a very substantial way on the well-being and adequacy of care of some of the most vulnerable elderly people to enter hospital today. The nurses (and doctors) have been recruited, disciplined and their interests realigned with those of the managers whose apparent sole preoccupation is 'throughput' in order to maintain efficiency and to control unit costs. This is not to claim endless resources from some 'bottomless pit'. It is, however, a plea that the proper study of the nurse at the end of the 20th century should include continuing analyses of the impact of organisational change, such as that brought about by health care reform, on nurses' professional behaviour and its impact on patients' well-being and health outcomes.

Certainly, some of our predictions, perhaps predictably, came true. Nursing, because of its ageing population structure and falling levels of recruitment, is becoming a smaller profession (ENB 1998), so much so that there is to be a campaign to recruit large numbers of students over the next few years (Cooper 1998). However, the economic notion that the price of labour should rise in response to demand has, until recently, not been seen to have any effect, for the diminishing number of nurses has not led to any relative improvement in pay. However, the Government's recent promise that the recruitment campaign is to be augmented by paying serious attention to nursing's worsening position in the pay league of public sector workers (Nursing Standard News 1998) has resonances with events in the 1960s and 1970s when nurses fell behind periodically only to 'catch up' when shortages threatened.

Finally, the research reported in this chapter contains salutary lessons for nurses engaged in interdisciplinary research. The *competing interests* of our subtitle have been more in evidence in this chapter than the *complementary interpretations*. As the project leader of the Griffiths research I was not always comfortable with the analyses which I and my co-researcher were developing. Nevertheless, gradually, I allowed myself to be persuaded to a particular analytic perspective by a researcher who was highly regarded in the academic world, and more experienced in that environment than I was at the time. Many of his arguments for the development of nursing were highly persuasive and, in the prevailing climate of opinion, our approach seemed more likely to benefit nurses than if we had been the bearers of bad news. As a result, we did not fully develop the analysis of nursing's continuing subordination, nor the decimation of its management structure which, arguably, diminished nursing's influence even more. The judgement as to whether our research made any difference to contemporary nursing has to rest on the available evidence. Undoubtedly, our campaign for nurses to address the issue of the cost-effectiveness of the nursing services will have contributed in some part to the progressive development of research on nursing which has been taking place in Britain since the beginning of the 1990s decade. That much of this research is now multidisciplinary within the overall context of health services research is, we believe, a very positive sign. Nevertheless, nurse researchers need to be ever vigilant that they are not being subject to the realignment of their interests by fellow researchers with the prestige and power to claim that theirs is the only true interpretation of the evidence. In practice settings, as Joanna's and Michael's chapters illustrate, there is still much persuasive (or harder-line) realignment going on. Nurses need to ask themselves therefore whether the managerial strategies to which they are being recruited meet the moral and ethical beliefs discussed by Mark Avis in Chapters 3 and 4, and whether they participate sufficiently in dialogues which address questions about the kind of society we live in, and the kind of society we ought to have.

REFERENCES

Aiken L H, Sloane D M 1997 Effects of organizational innovations in AIDS care on burnout among urban hospital nurses. Work and Occupations 24(4): 453–477
Aiken L H, Smith H L, Lake E T 1994 Lower Medicare mortality among a set of hospitals known for good nursing care. Medical Care 32(8): 771–787
Aiken L H, Sloane D M, Lake E T 1997 Satisfaction with inpatient acquired immunodeficiency syndrome care. Medical Care 35(9): 948–962
American Public Health Association 1997 Hospital restructuring in North America and Europe: patient outcomes and workforce implications. Medical Care 35(10) (suppl)
Cooper G 1998 Alarm over shortage of nurses. The Independent, 5 August, p 7
Davies C 1995 Gender and the professional predicament in nursing. Open University Press, Milton Keynes

Department of Health (DoH) 1989a Working for patients. HMSO, London
Department of Health (DoH) 1989b Caring for people: community care in the next
    decade and beyond. HMSO, London
Department of Health (DoH) 1997 The new NHS: modern, dependable. The Stationery
    Office, London
Department of Health (DoH) 1998 Our healthier nation. The Stationery Office, London
Department of Health and Social Security (DHSS) 1972 National Health Service
    reorganisation: England. HMSO, London
Department of Health and Social Security (DHSS) 1980 Health service development:
    structure and management. HC(80)8, DHSS, London
Department of Health and Social Security (DHSS) 1983 NHS management inquiry
    report. (The Griffiths Report) DA(83)38, DHSS, London
Department of Health and Social Security (DHSS) 1984 Health service management:
    implementation of the NHS management inquiry report. HC(84)13, DHSS, London
Department of Health and Social Security and Welsh Office 1979 Patients first. HMSO,
    London
English National Board for Nursing, Midwifery and Health Visiting (ENB) 1998
    Annual Report 1997–1998. ENB, London
Nursing Policy Studies Centre 1988 Quadrennial report 1985–1988. NPSC, University
    of Warwick
Nursing Standard News 1998 Blair agrees to talk on review body role. Nursing
    Standard 12(45): 5
Priestley C 1986 Promoting the efficiency of central government. In: Shenfield A et al
    (eds) Managing the bureauocracy. Adam Smith Institute
Robinson J 1982 An evaluation of health visiting. Council for the Education and
    Training of Health Visitors/English National Board for Nursing, Midwifery and
    Health Visiting, London
Robinson J 1992 Introduction: beginning the study of nursing policy. In: Robinson
    J, Strong P, Elkan R 1992 Policy issues in nursing. Open University Press, Milton
    Keynes
Robinson J, Strong P 1987 Professional nursing advice after Griffiths: an interim
    report. Nursing Policy Studies 1. Nursing Policy Studies Centre, University of
    Warwick
Robinson J, Strong P, Elkan R 1989 Griffiths and the nurses: a national survey of
    CNAs. Nursing Policy Studies 4. Nursing Policy Studies Centre, University of
    Warwick
Robinson J, Gray A, Elkan R (eds) 1992 Policy issues in nursing. Open University
    Press, Milton Keynes
Strong P, Robinson J 1988 New model management: Griffiths and the NHS. Nursing
    Policy Studies 3. Nursing Policy Studies Centre, University of Warwick
Strong P, Robinson J 1990 The NHS under new management. Open University Press,
    Milton Keynes
Webster C 1993 The National Health Service: The first forty years. In: Light D, May A
    (eds) Britain's health system: from welfare state to managed markets. Faulkner and
    Gray, New York

The World Bank and the World Health Organization: international sources of ideas for health policy

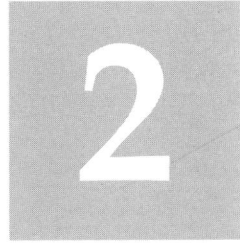

Jane Robinson

■ CONTENTS

Introduction   53
Competing ideas in
   health policy   57
The early origins of the two
   organisations   61
The policy process   63
   Case study: international
      public health   64
   Stabilisation of the
      world economy   66
Economic crisis and development:
   the background to health

policy developments after the
   Second World War   67
Responses to the economic crises
   of the 1970s   69
A realignment of ideas?   72
Conclusion: will pluralistic
   approaches to health care
   provision work in practice in
   the 21st century?   76
References   78

INTRODUCTION

On June 5 1998 a BBC report on the 9 p.m. news described Zambia's worsening health situation. Infant mortality rates are rising, and a nurse interviewed in a local health clinic reported that malaria is now the commonest cause of death amongst children, followed closely by diarrhoeal diseases. Infants, it was reported, are not benefiting from preventive health schemes. There has been no anti-malarial programme since the late 1980s, and as parents have to pay the equivalent of 50 English pence for access to the local health centre, many do not use it for their children until it is too late. The charge is frequently beyond their slender financial means. At the same time, it was reported that the Zambian Government is repaying three times as much in interest on its international debt on foreign loans as it spends on health care for its population. The implication of the report is that the economic dependence of one of the poorest countries in the world on developed world finance is driving the people into ever lower health status. Zambia, in 1995, had an annual income per head of population which was the equivalent of 400 US dollars ($400 per capita) (WHO 1998).

In this chapter, the theoretical underpinnings of the approaches to health and health care provision by two international organisations – the World Health Organization and The World Bank – will be considered in an attempt to trace some of the international influences on contemporary discourses in health care. In particular, the chapter will examine the background concerns with, on the one hand, social justice and equity, and on the other, with what are broadly described as utilitarian approaches to health care provision. These issues relate to the philosophical subject matter of Mark Avis's chapters (3 and 4), especially to the ideas of what is required for human flourishing, and what is meant by social justice, but they also lead implicitly to concerns over the construction of discourses and the realignment of interests which Michael Traynor and Joanna Latimer explore.

The chapter is concerned with some of the policy origins of situations of which the Zambian report is an all too frequent example, and addresses the question of whether the international community has learned from the lessons of history and, if so, what might the solutions be? It is argued that the policy developments which are implicated in the Zambian and other similar situations appear to be partly an effect of a drive for efficiency in the public sector, which includes the phenomenon of health care reform, currently taking place across the world. The chapter begins with a review of some of the policies of The World Bank and the World Health Organization which have been put into effect over the past 20 or more years. The chapter then reviews the two organisations' longer-term history to identify the origins of these more recent policy developments, using case studies of the development of international public health and the stabilisation of the world economy to illustrate how the ideas behind the policies were generated, supported by governments. The chapter then returns to the post-1970s era, examining the goals and aspirations embodied in the more recent policy developments of the two organisations and some of the unintended consequences which have emerged. The chapter concludes that, as we move towards the 21st century, the signs are that a realignment of ideas is taking place and that The World Bank and the World Health Organization are moving closer together in recognition that no one theoretical position on policy development can possibly offer all the solutions to the global crises that we face. As yet, however, there is no evidence that this new pluralistic collaboration will necessarily solve the problems faced by Zambia and countries in similar situations.

Chapter 1 described research undertaken into the NHS reforms of the 1980s to show how contemporary concern with 'efficiency', set within the much broader historical context of the introduction of 'managerial' methods of monitoring and control, came to provide a backdrop for the construction of nursing and managerial discourses in the National Health Service described in Michael Traynor's chapters (5 and 6), and the realignment of interests and identity explored by Joanna Latimer (Chs 7 and 8). Reference was made to the enormous sweeps of history which must be grasped in order to contextualise the political events which we experience today. Sustaining this grasp on history is, of course, something of a challenge for most people in the midst of busy lives. Health care practitioners are rarely also political or economic historians and so we rely on others to bring these insights to our attention. Yet, as was shown in Chapter 1, any version of events is presented through a particular 'lens' which may be challenged by arguments developed in the context of a different interpretation of the facts. The need for health care practitioners to be aware of and, if necessary, to challenge the often implicit ideas which drive contemporary health care policy is a major underlying theme of this book.

The origin of the 'lens' through which the subject matter of this chapter is viewed lies in my personal experience of working on several projects since 1985 for the World Health Organization, and of a secondment to The World Bank in Washington DC, in 1997, on a Fulbright Senior Research Scholarship. During the secondment I also went on a mission to Indonesia, accompanying a senior economist on a project designed to strengthen the health professions, particularly nursing and midwifery. This gave me the opportunity to observe at first hand how Bank employees *actually* work, in contrast to the more lurid descriptions which may be found in some accounts in the literature.

I had been fascinated for some time by the emerging importance of The World Bank in international health policy, particularly the publication of the *World Development Report 1993: investing in health* (World Bank 1993), and found the secondment a stimulating opportunity to observe some similarities but also the considerable differences between the ways of working of the two organisations. At first sight The World Bank (or 'the Bank' as it is frequently referred to) may appear to have little to do with the development of health policy strategies, yet it was reported in 1997 that:

> Bank involvement in the HNP (Health, Nutrition and Population) sector, which started in the early 1970s, initially helped countries strengthen and expand the infrastructure and supplies for basic (health) programs. Although modest success was achieved through this approach, it became apparent that institutional and systemic changes were often needed for a sustained impact on outcomes for the poor, improved performance of health systems, and sustainable financing ... Since its first HNP loan in 1970, the Bank's activities in this sector have grown rapidly to the point where it is now the single largest external source of HNP financing in low to middle income countries. Today, there are 154 active and 94 completed Bank HNP projects, for a total cumulative value of US$13.5 billion in 1996 prices.
>
> (World Bank 1997a, p. vii)

Further, the Bank states an enhanced commitment to the HNP sector during the period leading into the 21st century with the objective to:

- improve the health, nutrition and population outcomes of the poor, and to protect the rest of the population from the impoverishing effects of illness, malnutrition and high fertility;
- enhance the performance of health care systems by promoting equitable access to preventive and curative health, nutrition and population services that are affordable, effective, well managed, of good quality, and responsive to clients; and
- secure sustainable health care financing by mobilising adequate levels of resources, establishing broad-based risk pooling mechanisms, and maintaining effective control over public and private expenditure.

(World Bank 1997a, p. viii)

Gill Walt (1994) in an important chapter on the international organisations involved in influencing international and national health policy, in her book *Health Policy: an introduction to process and power*, describes the Bank's activities as a quite deliberate strategy to position itself both operationally and intellectually at the fulcrum of international health development (p. 127). Walt asks what influence the Bank, in assuming 'a more central role as a major financier and as an authoritative source of policy ideas', will have on the future mandate for health among the 'United Nations (UN) agencies currently involved? How will the Bank's involvement influence pluralism in agenda setting? What are the potential positive and negative implications for having a Bank at the fulcrum of health policy development?' (Walt 1994, pp. 129, 130). She concludes that the answers to these questions require further analysis of the relationship between international and national policy makers in health.

For reasons which are discussed in this chapter, this much needed analysis is extraordinarily complex and has hardly begun. News items such as the one reported by the BBC on Zambia referred to at the beginning of the chapter, tend to implicate international financial institutions, including the Bank, in their analysis of the responsibility for such major human tragedies. Greedy or corrupt western bankers are, it is implied, expropriating Third World countries' assets leaving the populations to the consequences of extreme poverty. How, I asked myself, could an institution which sets out such apparently altruistic aims as those quoted above in its terms of reference for involvement in health policy, become an object of major criticism as the instrument of a situation which is exactly the opposite of what it claims to achieve? Further, what is the place of the World Health Organization in relation to this analysis? We have become very familiar in the United Kingdom (UK) with attributing and supporting our beliefs in primary health care to the World Health Organization's philosophy of health for all by the year 2000 (WHO 1978, 1981). Why, when we are much less used to attributing some of the more recent developments in health care reform to ideas which have been derived from The World Bank's initiatives, does the World Health Organization suddenly have to be seen in relation to the Bank?

COMPETING IDEAS IN HEALTH POLICY

The interpretation which I shall develop is that for approximately 20 years during the two decades of the 1970s and 1980s, frequently incompatible sets of ideas were driving developments in international health policy, which in turn, influenced national policies. As Joanna and Michael's respective chapters show, these ideas continue to generate ambiguities in health care practice today over the 'proper' purpose of health care institutions. These sets of ideas might be described from an *ethical standpoint* as broadly utilitarian on the one hand, and concerned with social justice and equity on the other. Mark Avis, in his chapter on 'Social justice and the right to health care', discusses these ideas in detail. Summed up in the maxim 'the greatest good for the greatest number', utilitarianism has been appropriated in health economics to justify defining which health care interventions and activities will result in the maximum beneficial outcome for a certain level of input – the roots of contemporary concern with *efficiency*. The result of the application of this definition of utilitarianism to health care is that policy is determined not by individual expressions of need but from the calculation of benefit maximisation for the majority. The preoccupation with *ends* rather than *means* which has resulted from this interpretation of utilitarian approaches to health care policy is opposed by deontologists who believe that all people's lives are of equal intrinsic value, and that it is neither possible nor ethical to place a greater value on one person's life than another (Seedhouse 1993). The economic notion that it may be necessary to treat one person in preference to another because this represents a more efficient use of resources is anathema to deontologists who believe that the health care professional's 'duty of care' to each individual patient overrides any other consideration (Robinson & Elkan 1996, pp. 119–120).

There is, however, another powerful critique of the way in which utilitarianism is applied in modern welfare economics. Amartya Sen (1987) in *On Ethics and Economics* argues that economics evolved as a *branch of ethics*. Adam Smith, famously attributed by neo-liberals with introducing the idea of self-interest as the driving source of human motivation, and of the market as the most efficient way to conduct economic affairs, was Professor of Moral Philosophy at the University of Glasgow from 1752 to 1764 (Raphael & Macfie 1976). Sen develops a systematic critique of this popular interpretation of Smith and, also, of the practice of modern economics, suggesting that the ethics-related tradition of economics goes back at least to Aristotle. Sen sees two central issues in this relation between economics and ethics. The first concerns the 'problem of human motivation related to the broadly ethical Socratic question "How should one live?"' and the second 'concerns the judgement of social achievement. Aristotle related this to the end of achieving "the good for man"' (Sen 1987, pp 3–4). Sen continues that the 'ethics-related view of social achievement cannot stop the evaluation short at some arbitrary point like "satisfying efficiency"'. The assessment has to be more fully ethical, and take a broader view of 'the good' (Sen 1987, p. 4). Sen also describes the 'engineering' approach to economics which, he agrees, has solved many of the technical problems in modern economics. The engineering approach is, he argues, characterised, however, by a very superficial view of human motivation in which neither the Socratic nor the Aristotelian questions figure. Sen argues that, as a result, modern economics has been substantially impoverished by the distance which has grown between ethics and economics. I shall return to this issue later in the chapter.

From a *political economic perspective* the ideas of social justice and equity, and utilitarianism (as currently equated with notions of efficiency) have also come to be related to ideas of positive and negative freedom, and the question of human rights in health care. A major problem when discussing human rights is whether the right under discussion refers to an individual's right to freedom *from* the interference of the State, or another individual, in the exercise of free will and freedom to act in such a way as to pursue a good life according to one's own will. Or, alternatively, whether the right refers to the freedom *to be* protected or enabled by the State in terms of positive discrimination or affirmation (Robinson 1997, p. 10). The use of its power by the State to improve the opportunities of less advantaged members of society in terms of improving their health, education, employment status, or freedom from discrimination, has come to be known as the exercise of *positive freedom*, or the freedom to be enabled to participate in society. *Negative freedom*, on the other hand, implies that the individual is free from coercion, is not dependent on the arbitrary will of another, subject only to the rule of law (Green 1987).

Practical policies advanced by The World Bank and the World Health Organization during the period from the second half of the 1970s to the late 1980s were underpinned on the one hand by utilitarianism and negative freedom and, on the other, by the idea of social justice, equality and positive freedom. Unsurprisingly, they were often in mutually incompatible forms. However, because policy is rarely developed in a pure sense from abstract theories, the policies put forward also included deviations from, or confusions with, the original ideas. It was during the 1980s that the Bank began to become much more involved in health policy matters in the form of direct loans for health projects (such as help with the provision of clean water or sanitation). However, a considerable part of its influence on health resulted not so much from direct lending to countries for health projects, but indirectly through the economic policies required by the International Monetary Fund (IMF) as a response to increasing indebtedness in many less developed countries. These policies frequently required as a condition of a loan intended to restructure a country's overwhelming international debt, that substantial public sector reforms would be introduced. This resulted in a reduction of public subsidy to social welfare projects, to health services and to publicly provided education. As a consequence, because people's health status is dependent as much (if not more) on their socio-economic situation, these economic policies *in general* had a profound effect on people's health and well-being.

I shall suggest that the policies introduced during this period not only frequently failed to produce their intended effects but also had many unintended consequences. As a result, partly of great public criticism of these international institutions, a greater pluralism of ideas can be seen to be emerging in the 1990s, although some of the more extreme effects of the earlier era are still working their way through health systems. I see therefore the 1970s and 1980s as a crucially important time in which many tragedies occurred as a result of the implementation of policies which did not begin to take into account their possible unintended consequences, but which also gave rise to a massive learning experience.

This crucially important period in international health policy was preceded by another stretching back from the 1950s to at least the beginning of the 20th century. This was the 'modern' era in which a profound belief in the ultimate power of science and technology to solve the outstanding problems of health and disease influenced the development of health policy. The development of vaccines and the introduction of antibiotics gave the mistaken impression that for every health problem there was a potential cure only waiting to be discovered. In order to begin to unpack some of these issues it is necessary to go back to the early origins of the World Health Organization and The World Bank.

THE EARLY ORIGINS OF
THE TWO ORGANISATIONS

Both the World Health Organization and The World Bank owe their quite separate and unique existences to policy initiatives for rebuilding a world following the devastation incurred by the Second World War of 1939–1945, and both have their precursor developments in earlier times, in the case of public health to a century before. The origins of organised international public health are usually attributed to a series of international sanitary conferences, the first held in Paris in 1851, the purpose of which will be discussed below. In the first half of the 20th century, several international organisations were formed with responsibility for coordinating the prevention and control of (usually) communicable disease. Amongst these was the Office International d'Hygiene Publique (OIHP) established in Paris in 1907. A relatively small organisation, OIHP was paralleled in 1921 by an International Health Organization set up by the Council of the League of Nations following the ravages of the First World War and the breakdown of sanitary arrangements in many countries (WHO 1958, p. 29). Other bodies also existed, notably the Pan American Sanitary Bureau and the Egyptian Sanitary Maritime and Quarantine Board. By the mid-1930s the League of Nations had recognised the need to rationalise its complex committee structure, with special attention required for the Health Committee. The Second World War intervened, however, and this brought a cessation to collaborative international activities.

Immediately after the end of the Second World War in 1945, the United Nations was established to coordinate and increase cooperation between countries. In 1945 the United Nations Conference on International Organization also proposed that a single international health agency should be formed to deal with health matters. In 1946 the representatives of 61 governments ratified the constitution of the World Health Organization, as this new specialised agency of the United Nations was to be known. The objective of the Organization was to be the 'attainment by all peoples of the highest possible level of health' which was stated to be 'one of the fundamental rights of every human being without distinction of race, religion, political belief, economic or social condition' and to consist of 'a state of complete physical, mental and social well being' (World Health Organization

Constitution, WHO 1946). Thus the philosophy of positive freedom, social justice and equity, was written into the very foundations of the World Health Organization.

By contrast, The World Bank's origins lay in very different concerns for, during the 1940s, there was a grave fear amongst western economists and business interests that the world economy might collapse after the Second World War, thus repeating events which had followed the first. The global economic depression of the 1930s had resulted in individual countries introducing extremely damaging trade protection measures, repeated currency devaluations and the erection of trade barriers, which only served to drag all of the industrial nations ever deeper into a downward economic spiral. A profound need was therefore perceived to ensure the global economic order following the Second World War. In 1941, a Treasury official (Harry Dexter White) in the USA proposed a plan for a 'stabilisation fund' to keep world financial exchange rates in equilibrium, and 'a bank for reconstruction and development' to invest in countries damaged by the war (Caufield 1996, p. 40). Concurrently in Britain, the economist John Maynard Keynes who was serving as an advisor to the British Treasury, also had a plan for an international currency union to avoid the disastrous global economic conditions which had followed the First World War. In 1943, British and American officials met in Washington to discuss these respective ideas. The two sets of ideas were merged.

At first, 'a permanent institution for international monetary cooperation' (the International Monetary Fund) was proposed, but later at the Bretton Woods Conference convened in 1944 by President Roosevelt, the idea of an International Bank for Reconstruction and Development (IBRD, or World Bank) was also proposed and accepted (Caufield 1996, pp. 41, 42). The public case for the International Monetary Fund and The World Bank was that they were essential to the establishment of global prosperity following the Second World War (Caufield 1996, p. 49). Like the World Health Organization, The World Bank was formally established in 1946. The World Bank consists of two subdivisions, the International Bank for Reconstruction and Development (IBRD) and the International Development Association (IDA), whose functions are to make long-term loans at low rates of interest to least developed and developing countries in order to promote their economic development. The

World Bank *Group* also includes the International Finance Corporation (IFC) which lends to and invests in private companies, plus two further smaller agencies (Caufield 1996, pp. 66, 67). The IFC, in its role of development with the private sector, may positively encourage private investment in the health sector. The International Monetary Fund is a sister organisation of the Bank and exists to lend money to countries with severe balance of payments deficits, which, strictly speaking, is not the business of the Bank whose function is to lend money for specific development projects. However, in 1983 this principle was reversed and the Bank was allowed to make 10% of its annual lending in 'nonproject loans' in special circumstances to countries with balance of payment crises. A condition of these loans was that the countries would agree to reform their economies in line with the Bank's recommendations (Caufield 1996, p. 141).

Many of the initial statements of high ideals, and subsequent reports of problems of competition and leadership, and failures of organisation and intent, can be seen as recurring themes throughout the histories of both the World Health Organization and The World Bank. Hence, we do not see steady progress towards some supraordinate goal, or goals, but instead a series of initiatives which are more, or less, successful; are subject to more, or less, criticism; and all of which are built on influential individuals' (in particular, successive World Bank Presidents and World Health Organization Directors General) beliefs that a *particular* approach to a problem is the *correct* way in order to achieve the stated objectives. Looking at organisations in term of these policy processes can be a useful way to understand the processes whereby they function, their ability to influence, and their inherent weaknesses.

THE POLICY PROCESS

One way of appreciating these processes is to analyse why the policy issues which give rise to the initial formation of international organisations became of such *legitimate* concern to governments that they were prepared to lend the weight of their political and financial support to their establishment. Although to be of legitimate concern is *necessary* for an issue to reach the policy agenda, it is not a *sufficient* condition for action. The solutions advanced to address policy problems must also be seen to be *feasible* and they must have general *support*, not only from governments but also from a range of vested interests (Hall et al 1978). The feasibility of a proposed strategy is the 'wild card' element in bringing about change through organisational policy initiatives because the feasibility of a successful initiative is dependent on the current state of *knowledge* at the time the policy is made. However, the necessary knowledge may not exist or, if it does, knowledge is the subject of constant challenge and change and is superseded periodically by new paradigms to which a policy-making organisation has to adapt its strategies. There may not only be serious *political* objections to accepting the need for a change in policy direction if the new paradigm challenges the deeply held belief systems of those who hold controlling interests, but also it may be difficult *technically* because the new knowledge paradigm is not always easy to *apply*. If the organisation is then seen to be failing to meet its stated objectives, the support on which it is highly dependent may begin to weaken. In the case of international organisations such as The World Bank and the World Health Organization, this may lead to the organisation becoming the subject of overt criticism, the withholding of vital funds by member governments and, ultimately, to the transformation of its power base and, in extremis, to its demise. The following case study on the establishment, first, of international cooperation in public health and, second, in economic matters, serves to illustrate the points raised in this section.

Case study: international public health

The initial, tentative, development in the mid-19th century of an international organisation for the control of public health provides an example of the legitimation, feasibility and support for the policy processes described above. Cholera reached Western Europe for the first time in the 1830s. A combination of factors made this disease a terrifying reality for the countries of the western world. Cholera was no longer a hazard of spending time in the colonial empires of the world. Industrialisation, urbanisation, and the speed and facility of new transport systems meant that its rapid transmission could lead to the development of epidemics in any geographical location. Despite the wonders of new technology and the growth of international trade, an outbreak of cholera could threaten the stability of any government. The legislative action for the organisation of public health initiatives which began in Britain in the middle of the 19th century as a reaction to this threat, was accompanied during exactly the same period of time by the initiation of international efforts at collaboration. Public health initiatives thus became the *legitimate* concern of national governments and, through their concerns over disease transmission, of international significance.

The International Sanitary Conference held in Paris in 1851 is usually described as the first international attempt to organise in the promotion of public health, in particular to try to achieve some international consensus on the public health policy issues of cholera, plague and yellow fever (WHO 1958). The *legitimacy* of the policy issue was not therefore in question. The *feasibility* of doing something about it was, however, much more problematic. No-one in 1851 knew the *cause* of cholera, although the implication of polluted water supplies had by then been suggested, but there was certainly no treatment for affected persons. The only *feasible* international policy measure was the isolation of those infected, or potentially infected, if they were travellers from an area with a known outbreak of the disease. Hence, the outcome of the 1851 International Sanitary Conference was an international sanitary convention on minimum maritime *quarantine* arrangements, considered a necessity in the face of increased international trade. *Support* for this policy development (which was not universally forthcoming from all participants; WHO 1958, p. 10) was therefore strongly related to economic considerations.

This is a pattern which is frequently repeated in international cooperation in health policy matters. If economic benefits are unlikely to accrue to member states as a result of the particular health policy actions of international organisations, support is more likely to fade. The connection is not usually stated in such bleak terms. All democratic governments normally claim to subscribe to value systems which include the health and well-being of their peoples. Governments would be unlikely to become elected if they did not. As popular electoral support depends primarily on the voters' economic well-being, and if a healthy population contributes to this state of affairs, then it will be in governments' interests to support the achievement of the public's health (although different ways of financing and providing health services in different nation states will be proposed dependent on the strength of the political theories underpinning any particular government's actions). Nevertheless, there is almost inevitably a continued tension played out in the formulation of health policy. On the one hand, is its advocacy by those who argue that a healthy population is closely linked to a country's economic status and, on the other, the extent to which it is likely to be accepted by governments who will be lobbied by other interests less convinced of the strength of this relationship and more concerned about the probable costs. A continuing problem in resolving this dilemma lies in an absence of *unequivocal* evidence that the cause of the problem may be effectively addressed by any particular course of action. (Hence, contemporary concern with 'evidence-based practice'.)

Stabilisation of the world economy

The establishment of an organisation to stabilise the world economy was, by contrast with public health, *legitimated* by economists to lend money to countries in order to stimulate growth, and *supported* by governments and business interests who were desperate that the economic failures of the 1920s and 1930s should not be repeated after the Second World War. The *feasibility* of this initiative at the time was seen to lie in Keynes' economic theories of 'counter cyclical budgeting' (financing public spending at the low point of an economic cycle) in order to regenerate economic growth in countries devastated by war. Paradoxically, this theory was to be completely discredited when neo-liberal economic ideas came to dominate the world economy in the 1970s and 1980s and, as we shall see, the consequences then were for policies to be implemented which led to a dramatic worsening of the health status of some of the world's poorest populations.

It may be argued therefore that a fundamental difference between the two organisations lies in their underlying approach to health policy issues. The World Bank's loans to developing countries' governments in the health policy field are based primarily on the perspective of their *ultimate* contribution towards a country's economic development, a utilitarian objective. By contrast, the World Health Organization's remit as the directing and coordinating authority on international health work, is to *assist* governments, upon request, in the *process* of strengthening health services. Much of the World Health Organization's work in achieving its objectives is therefore technical and collaborative which, in turn, depends on the strength of the evidence on which it relies for its acceptance. It is notable, for example, that although periodic international sanitary conferences continued to be held throughout the second half of the 19th century, in the absence of scientific evidence to support the feasibility of further actions to prevent or to cure infectious diseases, no *permanent* international public health organisation was established. Once, however, the scientific problems of the epidemiology, prophylaxis and transmission of epidemic diseases had been solved, there were public health *applications* which could be managed and disseminated from an international agency. Hence, the Office International d'Hygiene Publique (OIHP) was established in Paris in 1907 under the auspices of 12 member states. The focus from the inception of OIHP (as with the later Health Organization of the League of Nations, the Pan American Sanitary Bureau and, the World Health Organization itself) was on the provision of information and advice relating to scientific and technical public health matters, particularly on matters of communicable disease, with interference in a country's internal affairs strictly forbidden.

ECONOMIC CRISIS AND DEVELOPMENT:
THE BACKGROUND TO HEALTH POLICY
DEVELOPMENTS AFTER THE SECOND WORLD WAR

Once established with their different origins and ideas as to process and purpose, the two organisations then focused quite separately on the problems of reconstruction and development in the respective fields of health, and economics. One view of the two decades following the Second World War is that the 1950s and 1960s were a period of relative optimism following unprecedented global conflict, the disruption of social and economic life, and the destruction of large swathes of the developed world's industrial infrastructure. As many industrial countries rebuilt their economies it was, for some, a period of steady economic growth. There was confidence in the growth of technical knowledge, both in the prevention and cure of disease and in the ability to manage economic affairs. During the first two decades of its existence the World Health Organization focused on limited technological interventions and on 'setting international norms and defining health care standards' (Peabody 1995).

However, as Walt (1994, pp. 123, 124) points out 'the vision of the United Nations overlooking a peaceful and secure world, supervised by a benevolent concert of great powers, was quickly dispelled.' The

United States had political, military, economic and financial hegemony. As the major provider of funds to United Nations agencies, the USA played a critical role in policy determination and, through the growing influence of the mass media, in the dissemination of the American cultural way of life. A substantial part of this dissemination involved a classical liberal view of equality (see Ch. 4), hostility to the communist powers of Eastern Europe, and mistrust of the social welfare policies established post-war in Western Europe. The policies which were most distrusted by the United States tended to involve the idea of positive freedom whereby states claimed to use their power and financial resources to offer forms of positive discrimination to improve the opportunities of the less advantaged in society. This notion of 'human flourishing' involves a belief in the participation of individuals in society, and health, education, shelter and employment are seen as necessary pre-conditions as a right of citizenship (see Ch. 3).

The USA, on the other hand, tended to support policies embodying the idea of negative freedom which involves the right of individuals to self-determination and non-interference by others, including the State. Apart from the maintenance of defence and law and order, proponents of negative freedom argue that it is up to individuals to make their choices and decisions about what to 'purchase' with regard to access to social benefits such as education, housing, employment and health care. Proponents of negative freedom argue that not only is individual freedom of choice crucial, but also that the competition which such policies produces results in far greater cost-effectiveness in service delivery. Thus, despite their ostensible non-interference in the internal affairs of member states, there were many subtle ways in which the agencies of the United Nations could be pressurised to recommend certain policies. This was particularly true in the case of economic development where the perceived need for less developed countries to industrialise and produce goods for export rather than subsistence, was closely related to the encouragement of private investment.

At the same time, many less developed countries remained colonies of western countries, only achieving independence after debilitating conflicts with their colonial masters. Their economic development was dependent on the belief that that they would benefit from a 'trickle down' theory of economic growth. Yet, despite their efforts to industrialise and diversify, many less developed countries remained in a dependency relationship with their developed world counterparts. They continued to export the primary commodities (which had made them so attractive as colonies in the first place) in return for foreign exchange earnings. The primary exports generated insufficient wealth to import manufactured goods, industrial supplies and agricultural technology to finance their economic development. Some less developed socialist countries (such as China, Cuba and Mozambique) cut off their links with western industrialised nations. This, they believed, was the only way to develop autonomously. Their health care models also diverged from the predominant western model and were characterised instead by low-cost, low-technology systems of primary health care. These were to become widely endorsed by the World Health Organization and UNICEF (United Nations Children's Fund) in the initiation of the health for all movement in the years following the global economic crisis in 1973 when OPEC (Organization of Petroleum Exporting Countries) first raised the price of oil.

A second oil price rise in 1979 resulted in a major global recession. Substantial rises in the price of manufactured goods, including petroleum, seriously affected all countries except oil exporters, and particularly the economies of less developed countries. At first, commercial banks were eager to lend the 'petro dollars' which were now in massive surplus and cheap overseas loans were relatively easy to obtain. However, by the 1980s, international interest rates had soared and less developed countries could not service the interest on their existing debts (Robinson 1997, pp. 13, 14). A large part of the history of The World Bank and the International Monetary fund in the early 1980s is concerned with how they dealt with the problem of maintaining the interest repayments of developing countries faced with these massive debts.

RESPONSES TO THE ECONOMIC CRISES
OF THE 1970S

The economic events of the 1970s had different effects on the policies of the World Health Organization and The World Bank which, in turn, affected national health and health services provision. First, by the mid-1970s it was clear that earlier optimism that less developed countries would in time 'catch up' with their first world neighbours had been an illusion. Writing of the time that the WHO/UNICEF Alma-Ata Conference was held in 1978, Navarro (1984) claimed that there were an estimated 800 million people in the world in absolute poverty; a third of all deaths occurred to children under 5; and 70–90% of people in the poorer countries of the world were without access to health services. In this view, high levels of infant, child or maternal mortality represent the negative effects of economic policies which have served to redistribute health as a result of a drive for competition and a reduction in the equitable distribution of social goods such as health or education services. If the poor are seen as unproductive members of society, then supporters of such policies may adopt a social Darwinism view, claiming that reduction in the numbers of the poor also reduces a potential drain on wealth.

The Alma-Ata Conference in 1978 resulted in the World Health Organization and UNICEF adopting a completely opposite perspective, endorsing the principles of social justice and equity in the distribution of low-technology, low-cost health care through the primary health care approach to service delivery (WHO 1978, 1981). Nevertheless, this represented an implicit abandoning of faith solely in the principle of continuous progress through technological development, and a recognition of the relationship between socioeconomic development, community participation and health.

Nursing in the World Health Organization took this mandate to heart and subsequent recommendations from the World Health Assembly (WHO 1983, 1989, 1992, 1996a), Expert Committees (WHO 1985a,b, 1996b), and Study Groups (WHO 1987, 1994) addressed aspects of nursing education and practice necessary for health for all by the year 2000. As a result, nursing world-wide began to reform the education and training requirements for the development of nursing practice which would be reoriented to primary health care approaches to service delivery. That the reality often proved to be very different had far more to do with the scepticism of many of their medical colleagues (whose training continued to be based on high-technology interventions rather than low-cost approaches to population health) than with any lack of idealism on the part of nurses. Yet, these are the origins of the idea of the first level generalist nurse, able to work in hospital or community, with specialisation following first registration, which has been developed in various ways around the world. As a consequence, nurses in many countries with minimal ratios of physicians to population found themselves as sole providers of health care, especially in rural areas or to the very poor. The idea did not stop with less developed countries but also was taken on enthusiastically by nurses in many developed countries of the world, although the extent to which their roles were expanded or extended was very much dependent on the controlling power of their medical colleagues.

Second, perhaps the greatest paradox of the effects of international policies on health during the 1980s was that whilst the World Health Organization was attempting to bring low-cost, low-technology health care solutions to the poorest countries of the world, one of the consequences of the intervention of the International Monetary Fund in managing Third World debt resulted in far worse health status for many of the poorest peoples, and less access to public health services. By the end of the 1970s many less developed countries were unable to repay the interest on the loans which they had taken out in more favourable times with the enthusiastic support of international banking agencies. Potential defaults on Third World loans at the end of the 1970s were huge. Caufield (1996, p. 137) reports that '[b]y 1978, one quarter of all money borrowed by non-OPEC Third World countries was used to pay interest on existing debt. The situation was particularly bad in Latin America, where borrowing doubled between 1976 and 1982, and 70 percent of new loans went to pay interest on old debt.' The situation where poor countries just borrowed more and more money simply to repay interest on existing loans brought the spectre of another global economic collapse, banks would fail and millions of small investors would suffer. From this situation was born the idea of macro-economic structural adjustment for countries which were deeply in unrepayable debt. The International Monetary Fund intervened with a package of reforms. In exchange for large loans in order to keep up the payments on existing debt, governments were required to cut back drastically on government spending. The overt intention was to 'halt inflation, gain economic efficiency, improve the balance of payments and promote growth by switching resources to production of "tradables" and through the unhindered operation of the market' (Ashfar & Dennis 1992, p. 3). The resultant cuts in public subsidies for basic foodstuffs, fertiliser and transport services;

reductions in government services in education and health; unemployment and increasing urbanisation as dispossessed rural workers left the land for the big cities in search for work, resulted in drastic deterioration in the health and living conditions of some of the poorest peoples in the worst affected countries. Alongside reported economic 'miracles' with massive reductions in inflation and a return to a balanced economy were also reports of massive increases in infant and under-5 mortality amongst the poorest sectors of these countries' populations (Navarro 1984).

A REALIGNMENT OF IDEAS?

Some of the countries of the world's integrated the World Health Organization's recommendations for primary health care into their philosophies for health care and their health services. But, as has already been described, many socialist countries already had community-based services which aimed to reach the majority of the population with primary and secondary health care services, and the social welfare systems of many Western European countries, particularly Scandinavia and Britain, prided themselves on their primary health care systems. However, by the mid-1980s the rather vague terminology of the World Health Organization health for all documents had come in for increasing criticism. Just as critics of macro-economic structural reform were pointing to the devastating effects on the health and well-being of some of the poorest peoples of the world, so critics of health for all asked whether the World Health Organization policies had made any *real* difference to the people's health. In 1985 the European Office of the World Health Organization led the way in developing 39 targets for the achievement of health for all which were designed to give some form and content to the somewhat abstract ideas which the policy had earlier embodied (WHO 1985c). The idea of targets for achievement was to be taken up globally, and eventually found its national expression in documents such as the British targets for the Health of the Nation strategy (DoH 1992).

But continuing deep scepticism concerning the soundness of the World Health Organization's strategies was spelt out at the Riga Conference held to review progress between the initiation of the health for all movement and the end of the century, held at the midpoint between the years 1978 and 2000 (WHO 1988). Later, speaking to the World Health Assembly in 1991, the Director General asserted that in a world faced with rapid and often unpredicted change, future health and social development would be crucially interdependent with the political will to bring about change combined with healthy economic development. Thus, the notion of some form of pluralism of ideas underpinning future global health policy strategies began overtly to enter the discourses of the World Health Organization.

By the beginning of the 1990s there was also increasing awareness on the part of the international community, and public concern regarding the complex interrelationships between all sectors of the economy and their impact on health. Writers on gender and development had drawn attention to the particularly adverse effect of economic structural adjustment on poor women and their children, and male domination of the economic sphere began to be powerfully challenged (Ashfar & Dennis 1992, Elson 1995, Joekes 1987, Moser 1993, Ostergaard 1992, Young 1993). A further major influence came from the report of The World Commission on Environment and Development, *Our Common Future* (1987), which reminded its readers, just as the early public health specialists had done at conferences in the middle of the 19th century, that the death and disease which follow environmental degradation, although weighted against the poor, is no respecter of persons. *Our Common Future* highlighted a series of major industrial and environmental disasters, including the Chernobyl nuclear reactor explosion, which had occurred in the middle of the 1980s as a consequence of the complex interrelationships between the drive for rapid industrialisation and technological expansion, and the absence of adequate regulation or regard for human and environmental effects.

The emphasis of the annual World Bank's World Development Reports in the 1990s also demonstrated a need to take into account the interconnectedness of all aspects of the economy, and the need to make special provision for the disadvantaged in any society in order to enable them to escape the worst excesses of their poverty. The World Bank World Development Reports on: *Poverty* (1990); *The Challenge of Development* (1991); *Development and the Environment* (1992); *Investing in Health* (1993); *Workers in an Integrating World* (1995); and *The State in a Changing World* (1997b), all emphasise to a greater or lesser extent the need for pluralism of ideas in their approaches to development. Thus, both the World Health Organization and The World Bank's public statements from the end of the 1980s onwards seem to imply a realisation that policies focused exclusively at either end of the spectrum of ideas, whether on social justice and equity, or on the economic idea of efficiency incorporated in macro-economic structural reform, had failed to deliver the hoped for reductions in poverty, or an improvement in the health of the poorest sectors of the population. By the middle 1990s the two organisations had entered into partnership agreements to work together in developing action for health development (WHO/The World Bank 1995, WHO 1995).

The World Bank's World Development Report 1993 *Investing in Health* epitomises these pluralistic approaches to the different strands of policy in order to bring about hoped for changes in health status. *Investing in Health* conveys three clear messages. First, foster an environment which enables households to improve their health. This will be achieved by addressing the problems of poverty, by promoting economic growth, expanding and improving education, and empowering women. Second, improve government spending on health by financing essential services to the poor which are of proven cost-effectiveness and which have demonstrable external benefits (for example, the treatment of tuberculosis or the provision of family planning services). Beyond the provision of these services, the Bank recommends that the role of governments in health care should be limited to regulation; improving the capacity of health insurance and health care markets to provide discretionary care. This regulatory function is seen to be crucial because of significant market failures arising from the high-risk nature of the investment. Third, the Bank recommends that diversity and competition in health care should be promoted. It points out that private, out-of-pocket, payments account for more than half the per capita expenditure on health care each year. Therefore cost recovery schemes through private payments, or the development of health insurance, are feasible beyond the package of essential clinical services. Although, the report notes additionally that studies on the effect of user fees are inconclusive and contradictory.

Contrary to my interpretation of *Investing in Health* as a move towards theoretical pluralism in health policy, Walt (1994) asserts that it brought together policies from the 1980s which heralded a new and proactive stance for the Bank in relation to national health policies and which allowed a framework of conditionality to be adopted in structural adjustment dialogues. She argues that the call for a diminished role for the State, increased reliance on the market to finance and deliver health care, the prioritisation of specific services, and programmes based on cost-effectiveness criteria allowed the Bank to adopt a comprehensive approach combining health finance and health delivery (Walt 1994, p. 129). Certainly, health services reform in the form of cuts in public subsidy, the introduction of 'cost-sharing' (a euphemism for the introduction of charges), increasing privatisation, diversification, and the devolution of budgetary responsibility and accountability to local managers matched by monitoring and regulation from above, has become a way of life in both developing and developed countries alike. Definitions of the term 'health services reform' may vary, as may the extent of the reforms themselves, but underpinning all the local rhetoric lie the notions of economic efficiency, value for money and control of public spending. Some of the language is borrowed directly from that of macro-economic structural reform, some from the new managerialism referred to in Chapter 1.

In Britain, it is predominantly the managerial/economic discourse which is now *legitimated* by health service managers on the grounds of diminishing financial availability, the growth in the numbers of dependent elderly persons, and rejection of the requirement that health care should provide anything other than essential *technical* interventions. Thus provision of health care, at least in the public sector, is *legitimated* again in terms of purely technical knowledge for which, increasingly, there must be evidence of *effectiveness*. This discourse is *supported* by governments whose objectives in a world of global markets are dominated by a need to achieve balance of payments stability and for whom public sector debt has become a totally unacceptable financial strategy. The *feasibility* of sustaining the managerial/economic discourse is seen to lie in the ability to monitor performance through data sources that are managed using increasingly sophisticated information technology. Together, the managerial/economic discourse which is generated tends to devalue the rather vague alternative discourse of social justice and equity derived from Alma-Ata and health for all. Yet, the question as Phil Strong would have posed it (Ch. 1) remains, is there evidence for these reforms of the benefits to health status and, if not, what are the alternatives?

CONCLUSION: WILL PLURALISTIC APPROACHES TO HEALTH CARE PROVISION WORK IN PRACTICE IN THE 21st CENTURY?

We come now full circle to the BBC report on health status in Zambia, recorded at the beginning of this chapter. Is this reported situation due to further exploitation of the poor, or is it an unintended consequence of international organisations trying to improve a desperate situation? There is no easy answer. But one of the lessons which I learned whilst seconded to The World Bank in 1997 was that making a loan to one of the least developed countries (say for the implementation of training for the delivery of family planning services, or an immunisation programme) over a defined time period, does nothing to answer the question: 'What happens once the loan money runs out?' Some countries have such low total per capita expenditure that they may spend annually less than $US5 per capita on health care. This can be compared with over $US2700 per capita spent in 1990 by the USA (World Bank 1993). Thus the issue of ensuring both an improvement in the country's *overall* financial capacity, plus the development of *sustainable* health programmes, has to be addressed. The situation of poverty and financial dependency may have arisen historically in the first place because of colonial exploitation, internal government corruption, or 'greedy bankers' (an issue which is reported to be alive and well today; Fay 1998) but hoping to 'put the clock back' and redress these past injustices is an illusion and will do nothing to improve the current situation. (Although ensuring that issues such as contemporary corruption are currently addressed by governments and not implicitly supported by the international community, is patently extremely important.)

What is known is that countries with similar income levels demonstrate very different outcomes in terms of the performance of their health systems. For example, there is a difference of 32 deaths per 1000 of children under 5 between Brazil and Venezuela, both of which have an annual per capita income of $US2800; and of 857 maternal deaths per 1000 live births between the Ivory Coast and Sri Lanka, both with an annual per capita income of $US700 (World Bank 1997a, p. 3). The World Bank admits that far more research is needed to understand fully the factors which influence this state of affairs, but clearly:

Differences in housing, access to clean water and satisfactory sanitation, education, income distribution, and culture all contribute to this variability, especially in low-income countries. But the use of knowledge about the determinants of poor health (eg. the links between maternal nutrition and low birth weight, hygiene and infections, and smoking and heart disease) and implementation of effective preventive and curative health care (eg. vaccinations, oral rehydration therapy, obstetric care, and drug treatment of tuberculosis) are also important in explaining these differences.

(World Bank 1997a, p. 3)

There is an undoubted need for detailed case study research on the reasons which lie behind the variations referred to above. However, one detailed study has already shown, following the examination of a range of factors implicated in the relationship between maternal and child mortality and diet, literacy, income, sanitation and safe water, and provision of medical services, that countries which emerge as *positive* outliers (Sri Lanka and Costa Rica) have adapted their health care development to their own unique conditions; directing curative and preventive services towards existing patterns of morbidity and malnutrition (Hertz et al 1994). By contrast, Hertz et al note that one negative outlier (Egypt) experiences a huge drain on its social development resources through the need to maintain a large military presence, in contrast to Costa Rica where the government had constitutionally rejected the right to have an army. So internal government policies for 'human flourishing' combined with the appropriate use of cost-effective health care can be shown to produce positive outcome indicators – a combination of the principles of social justice and equity and the mantra of the managerial/economic discourse. Not that the ways in which governments identify with issues, create a particular ethos, and prioritise their activities, concern health care alone. Conditions for 'human flourishing' require the wide range of socioeconomic benefits to which governments may (or may not) try to facilitate access for the poorest members of society. Such policies certainly have a ring of 'positive freedom' about them rather than the notion that, in a free society, individuals may use their freedom to make choices on the fundamental issues affecting health and well-being in their, and their families', lives.

The conclusion which I have reached on the desirability of a plurality of ideas in policies for health and social well-being may be seen as an undesirable attempt to 'sit on the fence'. Yet, the conclusions which I have drawn on both the practical and theoretical approaches of The World Bank and the World Health Organization suggest that as the 21st century approaches, both organisations are struggling to reorient their philosophies for health. The direction in which they are moving suggests that the two organisations are beginning to address Amartya Sen's contention that economics should not only engage in useful 'engineering' work, but also must return to its ethical roots and concern itself with the two fundamental questions of human existence – 'How should one live?' and 'What is good for man?' In the face of endless human frailty it is unlikely that Utopia will be reached, but as we leave a century in which the 'modern' has become 'postmodern' it would be no small achievement to return to these questions as a basis for determining the future directions of health and social policy. In the next two chapters, Mark Avis unpacks from a philosophical perspective some of the ideas which underpin the dilemmas which I have touched upon in national and international health policy. Mark addresses first, in Chapter 3, the issue of health needs and health care needs and in Chapter 4 the question of social justice and the right to health care.

REFERENCES

Ashfar H, Dennis C 1992 Women and adjustment policies in the Third World. Macmillan, London
Caufield C 1996 Masters of illusion. The World Bank and the poverty of nations. Macmillan, London
Department of Health (DoH) 1992 The health of the nation: a strategy for health in England. Cm 1986. HMSO, London
Elson D (ed) 1995 Male bias in the development process. Manchester University Press, Manchester
Fay S 1998 Greed is good… and it's never been so easy to get rich. Independent on Sunday, Section 2, pp 1–2
Green D G 1987 The new right: the counter revolution in political, economic and social thought. Wheatsheaf, Brighton
Hall P, Land H, Parker R, Webb A 1978 Change, choice and conflict in social policy. Heinemann, London
Hertz E, James R H, Landon J 1994 Social and environmental factors and life expectancy, infant mortality, and maternal mortality rates: results of a cross national comparison. Social Science and Medicine 39(1): 105–114
Joekes S 1987 Women in the world economy. Oxford University Press, Oxford
Moser C O N 1993 Gender planning and development: theory, practice and training. Routledge, London
Navarro V 1984 A critique of the ideological and political position of the Brandt Report and the Alma-Ata Declaration. International Journal of Health Services 14(2): 159–172
Ostergaard L 1992 Gender and development: a practical guide. Routledge, London
Peabody J W 1995 An organizational analysis of the World Health Organization: narrowing the gap between promise and performance. Social Science and Medicine 40(6): 731–742

Raphael D D, Macfie A L (eds) 1976 Adam Smith: the theory of moral sentiments. Liberty Classics, Indianapolis

Robinson J 1997 Sustainable development: implications for nursing and midwifery. Nursing/Midwifery Discussion Paper No. 1. WHO/HDP/NUR-MID/97.1. WHO, Health Systems Development Programme, Geneva

Robinson J, Elkan R 1996 Health needs assessment: theory and practice. Churchill Livingstone, Edinburgh

Seedhouse D 1993 Ethics: the heart of health care. John Wiley, Chichester

Sen A 1987 On ethics and economics. Blackwell, Oxford

Walt G 1994 Health policy: an introduction to process and power. Zed Books, London

World Bank 1990 World development report 1990: poverty. Oxford University Press, Oxford

World Bank 1991 World development report 1991: the challenge of development. Oxford University Press, Oxford

World Bank 1992 World development report 1992: development and the environment. Oxford University Press, Oxford

World Bank 1993 World development report 1993: investing in health. Oxford University Press, Oxford

World Bank 1995 World development report 1995: workers in an integrating world. Oxford University Press, Oxford

World Bank 1997a Sector strategy paper: health nutrition and population. HNP Family Human Development Network, The World Bank, Washington

World Bank 1997b World development report 1997: the State in a changing world. Oxford University Press, Oxford

World Commission on Environment and Development 1987 Our common future. Oxford University Press, Oxford

World Health Organization 1946 Constitution of the World Health Organization. Official Records of the World Health Organization, 2, 100, New York

World Health Organization 1958 The first ten years of the World Health Organization. WHO, Geneva

World Health Organization 1978 Alma-Ata 1978: primary health care. WHO Health for All Series No. 1. WHO, Geneva

World Health Organization 1981 Thirty fourth World Health Assembly Resolution WHA34.36. Global strategy for health for all by the year 2000. WHO, Geneva

World Health Organization 1983 Thirty Sixth World Health Assembly Resolution WHA36.11. The role of nursing/midwifery personnel in the strategy for health for all. WHO, Geneva

World Health Organization 1985a Education and training of nurse teachers and managers with special regard to primary health care. Report of a WHO Expert Committee. Technical Report Series 708. WHO, Geneva

World Health Organization 1985b Health manpower requirements for the achievement of health for all by the year 2000 through primary health care. Report of a WHO Expert Committee. Technical Report Series 717. WHO, Geneva

World Health Organization 1985c Targets for health for all. WHO Regional Office for Europe, Copenhagen

World Health Organization 1987 Regulatory mechanisms for nursing training and practice: meeting primary health care needs. Report of a WHO Study Group. Technical report Series 738. WHO, Geneva

World Health Organization 1988 From Alma-Ata to the year 2000: Reflections on the midpoint. WHO, Geneva

World Health Organization 1989 Forty Second World Health Assembly Resolution WHA42.27. Strengthening nursing and midwifery personnel in support of strategies for health for all. WHO, Geneva

World Health Organization 1991 Statements of Dr Hiroshi Nakajima, Director General, to the Executive Board and the Forty Fourth World Health Assembly. (unpublished document A44/DIV/4) WHO, Geneva

World Health Organization 1992 Forty Fifth World Health Assembly Resolution WHA45.5. Strengthening nursing and midwifery personnel in support of strategies for health for all. WHO, Geneva

World Health Organization 1994 Nursing beyond the year 2000. Report of a WHO Study Group. Technical report Series 842. WHO, Geneva

World Health Organization 1995 WHO and World Bank meet again to review progress in their collaboration. WHO Press Release WHA/5, 3 May 1995 (Forty Eighth World Health Assembly). WHO, Geneva

World Health Organization 1996a Forty Ninth World Health Assembly Resolution WHA49.1. Strengthening nursing and midwifery. WHO, Geneva

World Health Organization 1996b Nursing practice. Report of a WHO Expert Committee. Technical Report Series 860. WHO, Geneva

World Health Organization 1998 The world health report 1998. Life in the 21st century. A vision for all. Report of the Director General. WHO, Geneva

World Health Organization/The World Bank 1995 Partnership: recommendations for action for health and development. (unpublished document WHO/INA 95.1) WHO, Geneva

Young K 1993 Planning development with women: making a world of difference. Macmillan, London

Health needs and health care needs

Mark Avis

3

■ CONTENTS

Introduction   81
Needs and the NHS   82
   The grammar of need   84
   Needs are instrumental   84
   Health needs are relative   85
   Needs as universal drives   85
   No fundamental or basic
     needs   86
   Health economists and health
     care needs   87
   Health needs assessment   88

The postmodern turn   89
Rediscovering objective
   needs   92
   Teleology and biology   93
   Teleology and moral
     purposes   94
   A sketch of an account of
     objective human needs   95
Conclusion   96
References   97

INTRODUCTION

Service planning in the National Health Service (NHS) has been based on a model of identifying health care need, organising services to meet health care need, and then evaluating the success of those services in meeting need. The idea that meeting people's needs has an ethical dimension based on social consensus is captured by Titmuss (1987, p. 43):

> All collectively provided services are deliberately designed to meet certain socially recognised 'needs'; they are manifestations, first, of society's will to survive as an organic whole and secondly, of the expressed wish of all the people to assist in the survival of some people. Needs may therefore be thought of as 'social' and 'individual'; as interdependent, mutually related essentials for the continued existence of the parts and the whole.

Other chapters in this book, however, provide some evidence that need functions as a 'political' term (for example in Chs 7 and 8). The rhetorical force of revealing what is needed by patients is used by health professionals and managers alike to shape the development of health services, to legitimate their own activities, and to co-opt others into realigning interests with their own. Indeed, health economists such as Culyer and colleagues (1972) have complained that the idea of need is systematically ambiguous and corrupts policy discussion:

> the word 'need' ought to be banished from discussion of public policy ... in many public discussions it is difficult to tell, when someone says that 'society needs ...' whether he means that *he* needs it, whether he means that society ought to get it in *his* opinion, whether a majority of the members of society want it, or *all* of them want it. Nor it is clear whether it is 'needed' *regardless* of the cost to society.
>
> (Culyer et al 1972, p. 114)

Furthermore, there is currently a strand of political correctness that encourages a move away from the idea of need. Expert judgement about what others 'need' is merely a tactic to legitimate meddling in other people's affairs, and it implies that a person or community is in a state of dependency. It is argued that use of such a label disempowers people from doing anything about their own condition, and creates an expectation that others will 'do something' for them.

The purpose of this chapter is to examine how far the idea of need that Titmuss identified can be defended against more recent criticisms. The chapter will examine two views which call into question the idea of objective needs. First, a view that all needs are subjective and relative individual desires. Second, the idea that language and power shape what counts as needs. The chapter concludes by attempting to recover an objective account of human needs.

NEEDS AND THE NHS

Allsop (1984) suggests that five assumptions underpinned the creation of the NHS which, taken together, constitute an accepted understanding of health need: a *collectivist* principle of state responsibility for its citizens; a principle of *comprehensiveness* entailing a full range of health services 'from the cradle to the grave'; a *universal* principle that provided care free at the point of use; a principle of *equity* that set the same standard of service for all; and a principle of *professional autonomy*. However, from a philosophical perspective, Seedhouse (1994) has pointed out that an unquestioning acceptance of these principles as 'articles of faith' has prevented any critical examination of the political purpose of the NHS in social policy. Culyer (1976, p. 136) makes a similar point from a health economist's point of view:

Too many academic students of the NHS ... have tended towards the romantic view ... that the NHS, with its 'free' health care, is an end in itself rather than a means to an end. On the one hand this has led to an uncritical defence of the NHS ... on the other hand its [the romantic view] complacency has led to a void as far as real analysis of the NHS's problems are concerned.

The point is that without a clear statement of social purpose for the NHS, the idea of need which drives health policy is open to reinterpretation and reinvention according to prevailing political norms. Such a shift in political philosophy is detected by Klein (1993) in his observations on the managerial revolution that culminated in the 1990 NHS and Community Care Act:

> the new style and the new language reflect a different view of the health care system, a move from seeing it as a church to seeing it as a garage ... this process of secularisation is reflected in a linguistic revolution: the transformation of the patient into a consumer. The consumer is someone who goes out to satisfy his or her wants ... challenging the NHS needs-based distributive goals. The emphasis has switched from seeing the NHS as an instrument for promoting broad social goals ... to seeing it as satisfying individual expectations: specifically, expectations that people will get an efficient repair and maintenance service.
>
> (Klein 1993, p. 136)

In identifying the shift from viewing the NHS as church to garage, Klein seems to have captured a fundamental change in political rhetoric. Providing health care is no longer viewed as a social mission that requires an elite priesthood of health professionals who use their specialist knowledge to determine an individual or a population's objective health needs. Furthermore, a value system based on collective mutual aid is replaced by one of individual responsibility. The new rhetoric lays claim to an instrumental health service that uses strategies of rational economic management to deliver a service that gives people what they want. This is consistent with the evidence presented in later chapters by Michael Traynor and Joanna Latimer suggesting that the new managerialism employs a technical approach to problems such as meeting health need, using a strategy based on a rhetoric of measurement, moral neutrality and the efficient distribution of health care.

Meeting health need remains a central component in the presentation of health policy, but the monopoly that health professionals have had on the discovery of people's health needs, and the organisation of services to meet them is being challenged by the application of different discourses about the nature of need. The nursing response to this position uses characteristically moral language that introduces specifically ethical notions such as self-sacrifice, duty and rights. As Robinson & Elkan (1996) conclude 'most nurses believe that poor health implies a moral right to at least some level of care ... irrespective of whether such interventions are likely to prolong healthy life' (p. 224). Where professional norms of objectivity and service to others are being challenged by a new managerial rhetoric, the use of an explicitly moral framework by nurses can be understood as an important part of their professional identity work.

The grammar of need

My 3-year-old daughter has already understood an important aspect of the grammar of need. When I ask her to stop doing something she will often reply that she cannot stop straight away because she *needs* to finish what she is doing. She has recognised that need is stronger or more pressing than a mere want, and that it is linked to other longer-term goals. We can note several points about the nature of need. First, the grammar of need seems to imply that human needs are related to longer-term purposes. Second, a statement of need appears to be objective, whereas a statement of desire is subjective. When it is claimed that something is needed it appears to make an assertion about the facts of a person's condition, whereas a statement that someone wants something seems to refer to his or her contingent and subjective desires. Third, to say that somebody needs something creates an imperative or demands recognition in a way that to simply state that he or she wants it would not. The ordinary grammar of need implies that someone in need creates an obligation in others, a recognition that something ought to be done about his or her lack. This is why campaigners and policy makers couch their arguments in terms of need: 'we need more roads'; 'we need more hospitals', and so on. The concept of need carries considerable rhetorical force because of its implicit claim to be making objective statements. It is this feature of the grammar of need that provides legitimacy for professional and managerial activity in the NHS.

Needs are instrumental

We may feel the imperative for action created by statements such as 'Mr Jones needs his insulin'; 'Ward 13 needs extra staff'; or 'the District General Hospital (DGH) needs 50 more beds'. But such statements of need are incomplete. A need exists only when something is required in order to achieve some further, often unspecified, objective. The grammar of need contains the assumption that need occurs only when the means to achieve a goal are lacking. We can make this clear if we supply the unspecified objective from the above examples: Mr Jones needs insulin to avoid a diabetic coma; Ward 13 needs extra staff to manage the morning theatre list; the DGH needs 50 more beds to meet the expected rise in demand this winter. One of the problems with the language of need is that needs are often identified without reference to the desired goal; consequently we miss the fact that needs are a means to an end rather than an end in themselves. We can specify this point schematically: a person needs something when (a) there is a difference between his or her current abilities or resources and his or her goals, and (b) there is something that would enable him or her to achieve those goals. Once it is accepted that all need is instrumental, then it is clear that the moral imperative contained in the idea of need depends upon the moral character of the goal for which the need is instrumental. To have any moral force a need must be a means to a morally desirable end. Once it is clear that Mr Jones needs insulin in order to kill his wife then his need loses its moral force.

Health needs are relative

Once it is accepted that needs are instrumental, then it can be argued that any statement of need must be relative to a desire to achieve a particular goal. Need is *relative* to the desire to achieve an outcome for which the means are lacking. Therefore, the need for health is itself a means to a desired goal. Different people have different health needs depending on how much they need health in order to achieve their long- or short-term goals. People may need health only if it can get them down to the shops to buy a packet of cigarettes and a bottle of vodka a day. Others may need health only if it enables them to engage in other health-threatening activities such as boxing or scuba diving. Therefore, it can be argued that there is no universal need for health because the need for health is relative to the individual's desire to achieve some other goal.

Needs as universal drives

One alternative to an instrumental and relativist account of need is provided by Maslow's humanistic theory of need (1987). His theory is based on the idea that needs are drives to attain certain prerequisites of human life. He identifies five types of prerequisite arranged into a hierarchy of fulfilment. They are: physiological, safety, belongingness and love, self-esteem, and self actualisation needs. Indeed, it is interesting to note the central role that Maslow's account of universal and objective human need plays in the legitimation of nursing activity. It is difficult to underestimate the importance of his theory in allowing nurses to conceive of patients as having common and universal needs that legitimates nursing assessment (Lauri et al 1997, Yura & Walsh 1978). However, Maslow's account of need is unsatisfactory. First, there is no empirical evidence to support the claim that there are universal human drives that fall into the types he proposes. Second, his account of the temporal sequence of satisfying needs is simply false. There are many examples of individuals who pursue what Maslow terms higher level needs without having satisfied their most basic drives. Third, his account fails to provide an empirical link between the subjective experience of an urge to act and the instrumental account of human need required by ordinary usage of the term. It is simply not true that we always experience a drive to obtain the things we lack. It is not at all clear that Maslow's theory adds anything to the instrumental account of need, and it is empirically and conceptually inadequate to bear the weight that nursing theory demands of it. However, the extensive use of his theory in nursing models demonstrates the central role that the idea of universal and objective human need plays in the legitimation of nursing activity and its self-presentation as a moral enterprise.

No fundamental or basic needs

Notwithstanding Maslow's theory, the observation that need is *relative* to a desire for a particular goal and that people can have contradicting goals has some awkward consequences for professionals' claims about what people need. For example, a person with diabetes may have other goals apart from a desire to avoid a diabetic coma, such as an intense desire for a chocolate bar. Although we would hope that she places a desire to avoid a diabetic coma above the craving for chocolate, in the end that is up to her. What complicates the matter is that nurses may be tempted to assume that people with diabetes *ought to want* to avoid a diabetic coma. Therefore, it appears to nurses that a person with diabetes has an 'objective need' for insulin. The view that needs are instrumental and relative to individual goals requires scepticism with regard to claims that experts know what people need.

Critics point out that health professionals often fall into the trap of believing that people have fundamental, objective health needs because the professionals are using *their own* conceptions of the purpose of health and what someone ought to want. This trap tightens its grip on our thinking when we use specialised knowledge. Seedhouse (1994) argues that even something as seemingly basic as our need for oxygen cannot be taken as an absolute or fundamental need, because what is needed must change as an individual's objectives and goals change:

> Although oxygen is needed by human beings for most of the time, it is not always needed. According to our circumstances other needs might be greater … life may become unbearable and a person may need to commit suicide, and so choose to feed exhaust fumes into a sealed car. Reflection shows that any candidate for the title 'objective need' can be overridden as conditions alter and opinions change.
>
> (Seedhouse 1994, p. 35)

An expert, through the application of specialised knowledge, may be able to advise on the most efficient or effective means to achieve a desired goal, but an expert cannot judge what another person wants. This creates a paradox for the construction of nursing activity since, as has been noted already, nurses conceptualise their professional activity in terms of assessing and meeting patients' health needs. Once it is accepted that need is relative to the desire for a particular goal, then it can be seen that nurses' assessments of patients' health needs are more likely to be a consequence of their own professional purposes and self-identity rather than insight into patients' individual preferences.

Health economists and health care needs

If it can be shown that human need is instrumental, subjective, and relative to individual goals, then attention should be focused on the need for health services in terms of agreed health policy rather than as a moral imperative. As Culyer (1976) notes: 'the "need" for services … is in principle a technical matter which, while in practice is not devoid of the necessity for making judgements, does not require the making of *value* judgements about the ultimate ends of individuals' (p. 14). On this view, health care needs only exist when there is a recognition of their role as a means to achieve agreed health policy goals. This point is made clear in Culyer's rather startling example: 'Does the individual dying of thirst in the desert "need" a glass of water? Technically, yes, if he is to live. Normatively, yes only if others agree he ought to have it. If they do not, he may want it as much as it is possible to want anything, but he does not, on our definition, need it' (pp. 15–16). Culyer's argument trades on the notion that health need relates to the *gap* between people's resources and their individual health goals, but since each individual's health goals are personal and subjective there can be no general imperative to meet people's health needs.

As we noted earlier, the moral force of any claim about need depends upon the moral nature of the goal in question. Once it is accepted that individuals' health goals are subjective and relative to individual desires, then the idea of meeting health need is stripped of its moral force because there is no universal morally desirable health goal. As a consequence, health care need becomes a technical consideration relating to the efficient means to meet agreed health policy goals. From an economist's perspective, health policy should concern the best means to maximise health benefits for the population within the resources available. This may mean that the interests of the individual are subordinate to the interests of the majority. The point that health economists have driven home is that the need for health care, like any other demand, can and must be prioritised. We may have to meet some people's health care needs at the expense of others in order to maximise the overall benefits for society. In a situation of scarcity, decisions have to be made about which health care needs ought to be met and which not. The question of whether people ought to get the health care they need depends upon agreed policy, a view that conflicts with a professional, duty-based account of need.

Health needs assessment

The shift from 'church' to 'garage' revealed an underlying change in health policy, that it is concerned with providing the means for people to achieve what they want within certain socially agreed norms rather than providing what professionals think people need. Critics have pointed out that a health service based on what professionals think people need has led to an over-supply of some services, the provision of services that no-one wants, and a failure to supply some services that people do want (Stevens & Gabbay 1991). Current calls for needs assessment are supported by a technical and instrumental definition of health care need: 'an ability to benefit from a health care intervention at a reasonable cost' (Stevens & Gabbay 1991). This definition reflects an overriding concern with efficiency, and distributing health care resources to maximise the health of the local population within a fixed budget. It allows that not all health care needs can or should be met and licenses the substitution of cheaper, lower-quality alternatives and the trading off of health care needs against each other. However, a technical definition of health care need cannot obscure the lack of consensus amongst health planners, patients, managers, and professionals on the norms that inform the idea of a health benefit. It has been argued that a technical definition of health care need reinforces a biomedical understanding of health and illness, which marginalises social influences on health and healing and detracts from the need to consider the broader social purpose that underpins the provision of health care (Lightfoot 1995). The technical definition of health care need supports health need assessment that is little more than a method for determining the level of demand for a service that is defined by managerial norms and cash limits.

A genuinely pluralist approach to health need assessment should encompass popular epidemiology, which tries to enlist community concerns and lay knowledge about health and disease to seek political change (Mulhall 1996). Although critics suggest that these community profiling exercises are pointless, since without any extra resources to meet identified needs they simply raise people's expectations without any hope of their being satisfied, this is to miss the point of popular epidemiology, which is an attempt to influence the norms of local and national policy. We can see that treating health care need as a technical matter will only work if it can be assumed that there is consensus about the social norms that underpin the NHS. Changes in the metaphor for the NHS may reflect changes in the social consensus or show that the consensus is being contested.

The postmodern turn

I have suggested that the view of the NHS as a garage embodies a pragmatic and managerial approach to needs assessment which is in the ascendant in the NHS. This approach is based on technical concerns about the efficient distribution of resources. Such a view challenges the professional monopoly on the language of health needs and undermines a duty-based ethic that underpins professional notions of meeting health care need. Critics of modern managerialism such as Alasdair MacIntyre (1981) deplore the way in which a moral debate about human purposes and ethical goals has been supplanted by instrumental and emotivist language dominated by values such as efficiency, measurement, and technical expertise. On this view, NHS managers have attempted to secularise the language of need in order to subject it to a morally neutral and rational treatment.

Later chapters provide examples of how postmodern and poststructuralist analyses can reveal the role that discourses play in constructing our experience of the world, that discourse can be employed to make certain phenomena or social practices visible. Control of a particular form of discourse can be used to make claims about what is real, to exert authority, or direct social practices. In his many writings Foucault has provided accounts of the relation between discourse, the exercise of power and the conditions for understanding individual human needs (1973, 1977, 1982). A discourse structures social practices by 'guiding the possibility of conduct and putting in order the possible outcome' for the individual (Foucault 1982, p. 789). The exercise of power, mediated through the application of specialised discourse, organises the understanding that individuals have of their own needs and interests. The practice of modern medicine involves just such an application of a discourse to reveal objective and scientific truths about individuals, their needs and their possibilities for action. Armstrong (1984) uses Foucault's analysis to demonstrate how the subjective nature of 'patienthood' is constructed through the application of medical discourse. Social constructionists' accounts of need show that patients' needs are revealed by discourses that are themselves a fundamental feature in the realignment of interests. Such analyses of needs are persuasive since they allow us to see need as socially constructed by revealing the array of social practices and social contexts that support discriminatory judgements about human needs.

However, there is a difficulty in interpreting this analysis because it is based on a thoroughgoing epistemological relativism. Postmodernists argue that knowledge cannot be regarded as the progressive and incremental accumulation of facts and theories, but that knowledge itself is contingent and socially constructed. Human needs are not revealed simply by the application of knowledge about human biology, but are constructions based on contingent ways of thinking and talking about human biology. A postmodern analysis allows no truth outside a discourse, and therefore no facts about human need outside the application of a particular form of knowledge. Postmodernists provide compelling critiques of how knowledge, power and social practices are mutually constitutive, and how a discourse can be used to maintain authority and direct social practices. They do not, however, provide practical guidance on how we can escape from a particular discourse, or provide a basis for a better form of practice. In fact, as Porter (1996) argues, post-modern analysts are often silent on the matter. He points out that post-modern analyses cannot help us to improve our practices, in fact they deny the possibility of doing so because they do not allow that there are any facts outside a discourse to decide the matter. Although postmodernists accept that we can make judgements about the internal logic of a particular discourse, they deny the possibility of choosing between competing discourses.

MacIntyre's (1981) criticisms of modernism can equally be applied to postmodernism, that the moral dimension of the debate has become lost, and that the arguments of postmodernists are as rhetorical and instrumental as the modernist views they deconstruct. Many postmodernists and poststructuralists claim that an appeal to objective knowledge depends on the possibility of using science to provide what Rorty (1991) calls an 'intellectual skyhook' to lift us out of our contingent and cultural perspective on the world. They argue that the impossibility of this kind of objectivity means there can be no criteria that could settle disputes between different discourses, in which case we must accept judgemental relativism. However, this places the conduct of human enquiry in a false dichotomy; either to allow standards of objectivity that are acultural and ahistorical or to accept that all enquiry is perspectival, culturally and historically conditioned, and without common criteria by which to compare results. This overlooks the extensive common ground that is provided by everyday human language to conduct debate and seek consensus about what is true (Luntley 1995). I suggest that we do not have to give up ideas of objectivity or allow that where there are conflicting discourses there is judgemental relativism with no hope of settling the matter. On the contrary, as Rorty (1991) argues, engaging in rational dispute in search of unforced agreement is the defining feature of objectivity.

REDISCOVERING OBJECTIVE NEEDS

The first section of this chapter called into question an objective account of human need, and cast doubt upon the claims of professional nurses to locate their activity within a moral discourse of duty to meet patients' objective needs. The postmodern account provides an analysis that suggests that health needs are constituted by the discourses of professionals and managers, and that there is no objective fact of the matter to decide what patients really need. The postmodern analysis turns our attention to the moral and technocratic rhetoric that the nursing and managerial discourses respectively employ in an appeal to authority. However, I have argued that the postmodern account does not require us to give up on the idea of objectivity. In this final section I will argue that we can rediscover an account of objective need. However, it is not intended to be an account of objective need that 'trumps' all other considerations, such as political and economic concerns. Instead, it is an account of need that is objective in the sense that it provides a framework for dialogue about the nature of health care need within a pluralist context.

The critique of objective need given in the first section draws heavily on the idea that needs are dependent upon wants, and that what is needed is required because it enables us to meet our desired goals. However, this has the effect of 'psychologising' need. It makes need depend upon a person's beliefs and desires. It is compatible with a concept of need that relates to the means for 'desire-satisfaction', where the goal of public policy is to increase desire-satisfaction. However, this misses an important sense of need which we noted earlier, that need appeals to something objective. Need relates to a statement about a person's actual conditions rather than his or her state of mind.

It is legitimate to talk about needs without there being any requirement to attribute psychological states. It makes proper sense to speak of needs as requirements or necessities for an organism, organisation or a machine to function. Just because a person on hunger strike who is refusing food and water has no present need for them, or a suicidal person has no present need for oxygen, does not mean that human beings do not have an underlying and constant need for water, food and oxygen in order to function. In fact, it is only because there is an underlying functional need for water, food and oxygen that the protest of the hunger striker or the intentions of the suicidal person make any sense at all. This account of need relies on the function of an organism, organisation or machine. Such things need certain conditions for them to survive and flourish. It could be that one way of avoiding relativism about need is to start from a different point. Instead of trying to classify human needs in terms of individual goals, we should consider the purpose of human life and ask what needs humans have in relation to this. This type of explanation is referred to as teleological, since it derives from the Greek word *telos* meaning goal, task, or perfection. Teleological explanations attempt to account for things by appeal to their contribution to optimal states, normal functioning, or the attainment of goals (Honderich 1995). Aristotle argued that all living beings have an intrinsic tendency to develop towards fulfilment of their purposes or perfection.

Teleology and biology

Evolutionary biology provides one of the best examples of the applications of teleological explanation. One way of looking at the function of an organism is to see its purpose in terms of reproducing its genetic material. Dawkins' (1976) 'selfish gene' theory has revolutionised our view of individual organisms. On such a view, individuals do not act for the good of themselves, their families or their group but they act consistently for the benefit of their genes. If you think about it, every individual is descended from individuals who were successful at promoting their genes, and natural selection favours those individuals who adopt strategies that are most successful at promoting their genes. As Dawkins puts it, 'we are survival machines – robot vehicles blindly programmed to preserve the selfish molecules known as genes'. Here, then, is a concept of human need based on an answer to the question: 'What is the purpose of mankind?' Human needs are simply the necessities for the transmission of genes. This may seem to be far distant from the ideas expressed by Titmuss about the need for altruism to ensure collective survival. However, some new ideas in evolutionary biology have interesting connections with Titmuss' claims. It has been argued that cooperation and mutual reciprocation between individuals may, in fact, be the best strategy for promoting the transmission of an individual's genetic material (Ridley 1996). Evolutionary biology may show that the purposes of human genes are best served by altruistic behaviour such as mutual cooperation and reciprocal action between individuals. However, this does not help us explain the moral nature of human needs, only that the interests of genetic transmission may be served by mutual aid between individuals.

Teleology and moral purposes

Aristotle (384–322 BC) argued that human beings have an intrinsic tendency to develop towards fulfilment of their purpose, and he provided a specifically moral answer to the question of what is the purpose (*telos*) of mankind. Aristotle described the telos for mankind in terms of *eudaimonia*, literally translated as 'having a good guardian spirit' but which is usually interpreted as 'living a good life'. It is important to recognise that Aristotle's view of living a good life is an objective judgement. It is in contrast to a subjectively happy or contented life. Living a good life is not simply a question of having a good time, but of living a life to which others aspire. Aristotle maintained that an objectively desirable life is a matter of living a life in accordance with virtue. In common with many ancient Greek philosophers Aristotle held that the life of a virtuous person was intrinsically desirable, and that living a life of virtue aspired to a life in pursuit of human excellence (Aristotle, *Nichomachean Ethics*). Teleological arguments, by and large, have been superseded by scientific modes of thinking that place an emphasis on empirical and value-neutral descriptions of what is, rather than what ought to be. The teleological view has been further displaced by post-enlightenment and existential modes of thought that suggest that the purpose of mankind is whatever individuals choose it to be. In reply to these more recent arguments Alasdair MacIntyre (1981) has proposed that the displacement of the Aristotelian conception of the *telos* of mankind has left us unable to evaluate moral arguments about what is good for mankind. Consequently, we are left with merely technical answers to questions about human need that have become divorced from a moral conception of mankind's purpose. Amartya Sen (1987), quoted by Jane Robinson in Chapter 2 argues similarly to MacIntyre that the engineering approach adopted in modern economics has substantially impoverished the discipline by the distance which has grown between ethics and economics, resulting in a loss of the Aristotelian tradition.

A sketch of an account of objective human needs

Aristotle's teleological argument may provide the resources for a non-relative account of human need. It has to be accepted that need is an instrumental means to achieve a goal. However, the goal in question may be the pursuit of a good life or human flourishing. In accordance with MacIntyre's point of view we need to add that ideas of a good life and human flourishing are *objective*. Judgements may be partly determined by the historical context and culture of a particular society, the idea of human flourishing can be *essentially contestable* (Gallie 1956). However, acknowledging that ideas of human flourishing are contestable does not entail accepting that anything can count as an example of human flourishing. Wiggins & Dirmen (1987) argue that: 'ideas of life, harm, and flourishing are the focus of reasoned argument, and of a rich variety of opposing analogies, which it can still be hoped converge in agreement over essentials that is both principled and capable of justifying itself' (p. 63). Therefore, it is acknowledged that need is instrumental, but we preserve the objective, universalisable and non-relative character of need by setting out a moral and categorical purpose for human life that draws upon the idea of human flourishing. A person needs something in this non-relative sense if what is needed is a necessary requirement for pursuing human excellence, or good for mankind, or that without it he or she will suffer serious harm.

Doyal & Gough (1991) provide a fully worked example of how the idea of human flourishing and the avoidance of serious harm can provide an account of objective human needs. On their view, human flourishing is concerned with participation in society (this too has an Aristotelian character), and 'that health and autonomy are the basic needs which humans must satisfy in order to avoid the serious harm of fundamentally impaired participation in their form of life' (pp. 73–74). On Doyal & Gough's view, these basic needs are universal and objective because, whatever other individual goals and objectives a person may have, on a practical level, it would not be possible to achieve these goals without some degree of participation in society. However, there is also a moral dimension to their argument because without satisfaction of these basic needs the pursuit of a good life would not be possible.

CONCLUSION

I have suggested that the sceptical view that needs are subjective and relative to the individual allows the meeting of health need to become a technical matter about efficient distribution of health care resources. Second, I have argued that the social constructionist perspective on need highlights the way in which language and power shape the way we conceptualise human experience. This view calls into question the idea of objective human needs, since it regards 'need' as constituted through the application of discourses that serve, in part, to protect and preserve dominant social interests. If this is so, then professionals' and managers' claims to be organising their activities to meet people's objective needs may be a smokescreen for them to pursue their own interests. However, using a teleological conception of need that drew upon Aristotelian notions of human flourishing, I have argued that we can recover an account of objective human need that connects with the idea that there is a moral purpose to meeting other people's needs.

I have argued that although the concept of human need is contested, it cannot be reduced to a technical notion that can be made to fit existing expert or politically defined norms. The account of human need I have defended is objective in the sense that it appeals to a moral framework that provides the ground for rational dialogue. However, it is not intended to be objective in the sense that it trumps all other considerations, and even if we accept this account of objective health needs, there remain questions about the technical, economic and political means by which those needs could be met.

An account of objective need lends some support for a popular conception of a moral purpose for the NHS which cannot exclusively be defined by health professionals or by NHS managers but only by reference to a wider social consensus regarding ideas of human flourishing and a good life. It could be argued that the lingering popularity of the NHS, despite widespread criticisms of specific aspects of the service, is perhaps a reflection of the symbolic nature of the NHS (Taylor-Gooby 1992). It represents, as Titmuss (1987) noted, our altruistic concern for others who suffer misfortune, and the collective interests we have in cooperating and sharing in meeting other people's needs. This makes it possible to see the purpose of the NHS in terms of an implicit social consensus. However, the obligation to meet health need is being defined, and disputed, largely through the rhetoric of professionals and managers.

REFERENCES

Allsop J 1984 Health policy and the National Health Service. Longman, London
Aristotle 384–322 BC Nichomachean ethics. In: McKeon R (ed) 1941 The basic works of
    Aristotle. Random House, New York
Armstrong D 1984 The patient's view. Social Science and Medicine 18: 737–744
Culyer A 1976 Needs and the National Health Service. Martin Robertson, London
Culyer A, Lavers, Williams A 1972 Health indicators. In: Shonefield A, Shaw S (eds)
    Social indicators and social policy. Heinemann, London
Dawkins R 1976 The selfish gene. Oxford University Press, Oxford
Doyal L, Gough I 1991 A theory of human need. Macmillan, Basingstoke
Foucault M 1973 The birth of the clinic. Tavistock, London
Foucault M 1977 Discipline and punish. Penguin, Harmondsworth
Foucault M 1982 The subject and the power. Critical Enquiry 8: 778–795
Gallie R 1956 Essentially contested concepts. Proceedings of the Aristotelian Society
    56: 167–198
Honderich T 1995 The Oxford companion to philosophy. Oxford University Press,
    Oxford
Klein R 1993 The goals of health policy: church or garage? In: Harrison A (ed) Health
    care UK 1992/3. King's Fund Institute, London
Lauri S, Lepisto M, Kappeli S 1997 Patients' needs in hospital: nurses' and patients'
    views. Journal of Advanced Nursing 25: 339–346
Lightfoot J 1995 Identifying needs and setting priorities: issues of theory, policy and
    practice. Health and Social Care in the Community 3: 105–114
Luntley M 1995 Reason, truth and self: the postmodern reconditioned. Routledge,
    London
MacIntyre A 1981 After virtue, a study in moral theory. Duckworth, London
Maslow A 1987 Motivation and personality, 3rd edn. Harper and Row, New York
Mulhall A 1996 Epidemiology, nursing and healthcare: a new perspective. Macmillan,
    Basingstoke
NHS and Community Care Act 1990 HMSO, London
Porter S 1996 Real bodies, real needs: a critique of the application of Foucault's
    philosophy to nursing. Social Sciences in Health 2: 218–227
Ridley M 1996 The origins of virtue. Viking, London
Robinson J, Elkan R 1996 Health needs assessment: theory and practice. Churchill
    Livingstone, Edinburgh
Rorty R 1991 Objectivity, relativism, and truth. Cambridge University Press,
    Cambridge
Seedhouse D 1994 Fortress NHS: a philosophical review of the National Health
    Service. John Wiley, Chichester
Sen A 1987 On ethics and economics. Blackwell, Oxford
Stevens A, Gabbay J 1991 Needs assessment needs assessment. Health Trends 23:
    20–23
Taylor-Gooby P 1992 Attachment to the Welfare State. In: Jowell R, Brook L, Taylor B,
    Prior G (eds). British social attitudes: the 9th report. Dartmouth, Andover

Titmuss R 1987 The social division of welfare: some reflections on the search for equity. In: Abel-Smith B, Titmuss K (eds) The philosophy of welfare: selected writings of Richard M Titmuss. Allen and Unwin, London

Wiggins D, Dirmen S 1987 Needs, need, needing. Journal of Medical Ethics 13: 62–68

Yura H, Walsh M 1978 Human needs and the nursing process. Appleton-Century-Crofts, New York

Social justice and the right to health care

Mark Avis

4

■ CONTENTS

Introduction   99
Equality   100
Rights and duties   102
The 'visibility' of needs   105
Theories of social justice   106
   Utilitarian theory   106
Egalitarian theory   110
Entitlement theory   113
Individualism and
   social justice   114
Conclusion   115
References   117

INTRODUCTION

Health economists point out that in situations where there are limited health care resources difficult choices must be made between competing claims on those resources. In the National Health Service (NHS), where resources are fixed, providing treatment for some patients will mean that others miss out, termed an opportunity cost. This can be illustrated by the recent case of a child who was denied a specialised treatment for leukaemia, summarised by Watson (1997, p. 130).

> Recent public anguish about the case of Jaymee Bowen (Child B), who died from leukaemia in May 1996, is indicative of this problem. In March 1995 the Court of Appeal endorsed the decision by Cambridge Health Authority to deny Child B further chemotherapy and a second bone marrow transplant. Initially treatment has been withheld on the grounds that the probability of success was very slight and far outweighed by the trauma and suffering further intervention entailed. However, in his final judgement, Sir Thomas Bingham argued that the decision could also be justified on rationing criteria. The cost of the treatment denied amounted to some £75,000, and, it was argued, given the low prospects for success and the poor quality of life for Child B, it would be better to spend this sum meeting the needs of other patients.

This decision about the allocation of NHS resources would suggest that Jaymee Bowen's right to health care depended upon norms about acceptable quality of life and the opportunity costs of her treatment seen in the context of local health policy objectives. Since the availability of NHS resources for distribution to individuals depends upon a broad agreement about how much of our collective social wealth we are prepared to devote to health care, any right to health care is influenced by a consensus about the level of social resources we think ought to be dedicated to health care. The question of whether we ought to increase the amount of health care available involves consideration of the role of the NHS in promoting social justice.

Social justice concerns the distribution of social benefits in society. Social benefits include civil and legal rights, authority, property, education, health care, and social position. Social benefits go hand in hand with social burdens such as taxation and a reciprocal obligation to others. Questions about the distribution of social benefits concern the nature of a *fair* society, and the extent to which we are obliged to redistribute resources in society to counteract inequalities that result from chance and misfortune. As Gloucester says to his son, Edgar, disguised as the beggar Poor Tom in King Lear: 'Here, take this purse, thou whom the heavens plagues Have humbled to all strokes ... So distribution should undo excess, and each man have enough' (Shakespeare, King Lear, Act 4, Scene 1).

In the first half of this chapter I will examine the principle of equality and the notion of the right to health care to see whether either will provide a guide to the distribution of limited health care resources to individuals who need treatment. In the second half of the chapter I will review the three main theories of social justice in relation to the idea of a right to health care, and question whether any of them will support the redistribution of social resources to increase the amount of health care resources available.

EQUALITY

One conventional starting point for understanding the concept of social justice concerns the nature of equality. The classical liberal view of equality holds that in private life each person should be free to pursue his or her own interests without interference, providing they do not infringe the rights of others or inflict harm upon the wider public. This formal principle of equality is not primarily about a distribution of social benefits at all, but simply a recognition of equal protection for individual rights. However, there is a long tradition of conservative thought that denies that there is more to social justice than the formal principle of equality. This tradition rejects the priority of social goals and purposes over and above individual preferences. If social and economic inequality are the result of free and legal transactions between individuals who respect each other's rights then surely there can be no moral objection or reason to intervene to redistribute resources in society? However, a formal principle of equality may not be what people have in mind when they call for a fairer society. For many, a fair society should have what Nagel (1979) refers to as 'equality in the possession of benefits in general.' A distributive principle of equality plays a part in the traditions of socialist and reforming liberal thought that hold that all individuals need to share equally in the successes of society. One reason to favour a more comprehensive version of equality, one that aims for a fairer distribution of social benefits, is because life's lottery does not allocate physical, mental, social and financial resources to people equally. It can be argued that these differences between the most and the least fortunate should be taken into account in matters of rights and entitlements in a fair society. For example, equal access to health care does not amount to a fair system of distributing health care if it does not include consideration of the different needs of the individual. We would not consider it fair that someone who needs a minor operation for a non-life-threatening condition should have the same access to health care and be given the same priority as someone who needs urgent treatment for a life-threatening condition. Similarly, it could be argued that the current policy for distributing Child Benefit in the UK (a fixed benefit paid to the mother of each child up to the age of 16 years) is not fair precisely because it distributes the same resources to families based on the number of children they have irrespective of any other differences in their life circumstances.

It is important to differentiate between equality and impartiality. Clause 7 of the United Kingdom Central Council for Nurses, Midwives and Health Visitors (UKCC) Code of Professional Conduct (1992) requires each nurse to 'recognise and respect the uniqueness and individuality of each patient and client, and respond to their need for care, irrespective of their ethnic origin, religious beliefs, personal attributes, the nature of their health problems or any other factor'. Although this principle of impartiality draws upon the formal definition of equality that holds that each person's interests should be respected, it is consistent with a distributive principle of equality that attempts to achieve a fairer distribution of social benefits by treating people differently. One definition of equality that recognises the differences between people and which supports the notion of differential treatment is derived from Aristotle (384–322 BC). His definition can be summarised as follows: equals should be treated equally and unequals should be treated unequally. This principle of distributive equality is captured succinctly by Campbell et al (1997): 'people are treated in as fair a manner as possible by ignoring irrelevant differences between them but taking account of relevant differences' (p. 184). This account of equality preserves the importance of impartiality by requiring us to ignore morally irrelevant differences, which may include, depending on the particular issue, differences in ethnic origin, religious beliefs, sexual preference, and so on, but it recognises that equality does not mean treating everyone the same. However, it does not tell us which morally relevant differences between people should determine whether to treat them the same or differently. In trying to achieve a fair distribution of social benefits, including health care, one difference that could provide a criterion by which to discriminate between people would be their level of need. A fair society would aim for a distribution of social benefits based on individuals' needs. This is captured in the aphorism attributed to Marx: 'From each according to his ability; to each according to his need.'

Although different levels of need may provide a basis for discriminating between individuals in the interests of distributive equality, that leaves unanswered questions concerning the moral justification for redistributing resources in favour of those in need. To what extent do we have a social obligation to make individual sacrifices and give up our own resources through taxation or charity to meet the needs of others? Although different levels of need may provide a criterion for discriminating between people, this does not tell us whether we ought to meet their health care needs, or whether they have a right to have their health care needs met.

RIGHTS AND DUTIES

In the previous chapter we identified an account of objective human needs that drew upon preconditions for human flourishing. This account of need may give us some reason to think that some human needs are important enough to impose a duty on people to assist in their satisfaction. It has been claimed that these basic human needs are so fundamental that they have, by definition, a *right* to satisfaction. As Thomas Aquinas (1224/5–1274) wrote:

> Now, according to the natural order instituted by divine providence, material goods are provided for the satisfaction of human needs. Therefore, the division and appropriation of property, which proceeds from human law, must not hinder the satisfaction of man's necessity from such goods. Equally, whatever a man has in superabundance is owed, of natural right, to the poor for their sustenance.
>
> (Clark 1972, p. 384)

Starting from a very different point of view but arguing towards a similar conclusion, Robinson & Elkan (1996), drawing upon Doyal & Gough's (1991) theory of human need, say that: 'there is a moral imperative to meet fundamental human needs. The two basic needs for health and autonomy are not only the pre-requisites for participation in society, they are fundamental *rights* of all human beings.' The sense of moral outrage that often accompanies cases of children refused medical treatment provides some evidence of the widespread belief that we owe a duty of care to sick members of our society, and that the sick have a right to medical care.

The language of human rights, like the language of need, is fanned by political rhetoric, and often generates heat without any illumination. Rights, like needs, are attractive political counters in bargaining for entitlements since they appear to refer to objective properties. The idea of a human right is grounded in the moral duties owed to persons in recognising their individual interests and to accord them their full human dignity. In this sense, a moral right is the claim that a person's important interests ought to be protected. Put this way, it would appear that rights and duties can be mutually defined. Some writers have used this mutual dependence between rights and duties to make a distinction between negative and positive rights. Thompson et al (1994) put this succinctly:

> Rights which require people to desist from doing certain things to us, we call *negative rights*; and rights which entitle us to ask, or in some cases demand, that people do certain things for us we call *positive rights*. In this sense rights impose on others *duties to do things for us*, or *duties not to do things to us*.
>
> (Thompson et al, p. 90)

Jane Robinson has also discussed this perspective on human rights in Chapter 2 in the context of the different philosophies which have underpinned the policies of The World Bank and the World Health Organization.

However, the status of a positive right is unclear. The claim that a person has a right to assistance is an attempt to point out to others that they owe him or her a duty of beneficence. Most people would accept that they have a duty to help an injured person who they discover in the street. However, a passer-by may also have other serious and pressing moral concerns that override a duty of beneficence to the injured person. Consequently, it is not at all clear what is meant by the claim that the injured person has a positive right to a passer-by's assistance. In the absence of a reciprocal agreement that gives substance to the idea of a right to assistance, we must be careful not to assume that wherever a duty of beneficence exists, such as the obligation to help someone in need, there is a corresponding right to be helped.

This issue of a positive right to assistance is particularly pertinent for nurses, since their professional self-identity rests upon recognition of their role as instruments of a social consensus about the duty to assist those in need of health care. The importance of a reciprocal agreement as a basis for a positive right is demonstrated in Arthur's (1997) example of the duty of a lifeguard and the rights of a drowning swimmer.

> Here there is a clear sense in which the drowning victim may claim a right to have another do his utmost to save him. An agreement was reached whereby the lifeguard accepted the responsibility for the victim's welfare. The guard, in a sense, took on the goals of the swimmer as his own. To fail to aid is a special sort of injustice that the passer-by does not do. It seems clearly appropriate to speak of the lifeguard's failure to act as a case of a right being violated.
>
> (Arthur 1997, p. 601)

In a similar way, many nurses see their professional role as constituted through a general agreement with the rest of society which obliges them to take responsibility for their patients' welfare, and that their patients have a corresponding right to be helped. However, nurses' interpretation of the agreement that exists between them and society is subject to conflicting discourses about the duty of care and the right to receive care. This poses problems for NHS nurses in particular because the moral traditions of benevolence and self-sacrifice in nursing may conflict with a more utilitarian conception of social justice held by health service managers. Michael Traynor identifies these very conflicts at work in new NHS trusts in his research reported in Chapters 5 and 6, although they clearly do not owe their origin to the 1991 reforms. Robinson & Elkan (1996) put the two notions into sharp relief:

> nurses believe that they have an ethical 'duty of care'. They believe that as a society we should care for all those in need. Many economists, by contrast are utilitarians. They believe there is an ethical imperative to implement only those health care services which are expected to lead to best outcomes ... Nurses ... believe that there is something wrong with a health service which pursues only [these] outcomes to the extent of ignoring the actual suffering of real people.
>
> (Robinson & Elkan, p. 223)

THE 'VISIBILITY' OF NEEDS

This conflict becomes more complex when we consider how the application of a discourse can make certain health care needs 'visible'. Joanna Latimer provides a detailed account of how a 'translation of interests' in nursing results in a particular construction of patients' needs that makes patients suitable for processing efficiently. The significant feature of this process is captured by her descriptions of nurses' talk about assessing a patient's need 'by looking'. Moral disagreements about the allocation of health care resources will be constituted, in part, by the visibility of an individual's needs, and the visibility of the opportunity costs of meeting one individual's needs rather than those of another. As Watson (1997) notes, the media coverage of the Jaymee Bowen case ensured that the consequences of the failure to obtain treatment for the family of Jaymee Bowen were widely discussed, but the consequences for the unknown individuals who would have been denied immediate treatment if the treatment for Jaymee had gone ahead were unrecognised and all but invisible. This complication over the recognition of opportunity costs is particularly difficult because it depends upon the 'visibility' of the need for care. There is an opportunity for nurses, other health professionals, and health service managers to find themselves in conflict with each other over whose needs ought to be met as a result of the different perspectives on the visibility of patients' needs. Furthermore, professionals' recognition of a duty of care to the individuals they are treating may clash with a utilitarian perspective of health service managers who are concerned with the opportunity costs of decisions. These conflicting discourses are not easily resolved because a wider social agreement regarding policy objectives for the NHS in relation to social justice is lacking. Nurses' beliefs about their duty of care and their patients' reciprocal rights to assistance need to be considered in relation to their assumptions about a wider social consensus about the policy objectives of the NHS. Whether there is a consensus about the policy objectives of the NHS is open to question, and any interpretation of the policy objectives for the NHS will be contested by different concepts of social justice.

THEORIES OF SOCIAL JUSTICE

The idea of a fair society includes a distributive principle of equality based on recognition of unequal levels of need, but this principle cannot settle how much of society's resources ought to be committed to health care, nor how to decide between competing claims for health care. At least three competing principles of social justice can be identified, each of which could be used to determine a distribution of health care resources. The principles are, respectively, that distributions should be made according to social utility, according to human rights, or according to an individual's just desserts.

Utilitarian theory

Utilitarians do not separate a principle of distributive justice from a general ethical theory that we ought to act in ways that maximise overall social utility. Utilitarian theory holds that it is our moral duty to act for 'the greatest good for the greatest number' or the greatest benefit of all; and the moral character of policies and actions is judged according to the degree to which this outcome is secured. Therefore the utilitarian approach to social justice would consider that the best distribution of social benefits is that which maximises utility. The concept of utility may be construed in a number of different ways: classical utilitarians treat utility as net individual happiness or pleasure; more recent understandings of utility have tended towards regarding it as net individual preference-satisfaction. It is important to bear in mind that utilitarians treat each individual as a locus of value, and the present subjective preferences of each individual are the basis for the calculation of overall net utility. Consequently, the distinctiveness of each individual preference is outweighed by the aggregate of individual preferences. Utilitarianism is broadly equitable in the sense that each person is to count for one and no-one counts for more than one and, given that there will be a substantial number of preferences that people have in common, it is claimed that maximising utility will generally favour distributive equality (Nagel 1979). Although utilitarianism has fallen out of favour as a moral theory to govern personal behaviour, Goodin (1995) argues that the 'strength of utilitarianism, the problem to which it is a truly compelling solution, is as a guide to public rather than private conduct' (p. 8).

Several features of utilitarianism have attracted criticism. It is regarded as an impersonal *decision-making* where the moral agent is expected to take a neutral view in isolation from his or her social context and commitments. It has been regarded as a coldly *calculating* ethic based on an instrumental account of ethical behaviour. The only moral consideration is whether the action is effective in increasing utility, whereas the moral character of both the action and the actor are treated as irrelevant. Finally, the *crassness* of the nature of utility has been condemned. Utility, whether it is regarded as hedonistic pleasure maximisation or the aggregate of individual preference-satisfaction, seems to be weighted against the pursuit of aesthetic goals or higher concerns. Therefore, there are several good reasons to reject utilitarianism as a code of individual conduct. However, Goodin argues that most of these criticisms are virtues when considered as guides to public policy-making.

Nevertheless, the idea of utility as the ethical goal of human activity remains a central problem. The difficulty is that modern versions of utility, such as preference-satisfaction, depend upon individuals' current knowledge and subjective perception of their situation and, as such, these preferences can be manipulated by socialisation, advertising, and the exercise of power. As Lukes (1974) recognises in his account of power: 'To put the matter sharply A may exercise power over B by getting him to do what he does not want to do, but he also exercises power over him by influencing, shaping or determining his very wants' (p. 23). Utilitarians can be accused of legitimating paternalistic public policy, benign or otherwise, if utility cannot distinguish between the satisfaction of manipulated preferences and needs.

Furthermore, preferences can be regarded as adaptive, in the sense that individuals can adapt their preferences to those that are easily satisfied, at the expense of longer-term, difficult-to-satisfy preferences. If utilitarians attempt to respond to these objections by allowing utility to be defined by all *possible* preferences that people could have, they run the risk of being charged with paternalism again, because utility will depend upon the satisfaction of preferences that people ought to have.

Apart from paternalism, two central difficulties for a utilitarian view of social justice can be identified. First, it is clear that an individual claim to particular social benefits such as health care, property or civil rights can only be justified in so far as it maximises net social utility. Human rights can only be supported in so far as they are a necessary means to maximising utility, rather than an end in themselves. Jeremy Bentham, one of the founders of utilitarianism, is famous for his aphorism: 'natural rights is a simple nonsense: natural and impre-scriptible rights, rhetorical nonsense – nonsense on stilts' (Bentham 1843, p. 53). This is a serious problem for utilitarians since they do not treat human rights as intrinsically valuable.

The other concern that people express about utilitarian distribu-tions of social benefits is that they cannot, in principle, exclude patently unfair distributions of social benefits. Overall social utility may be increased if all people over the age of 85 were denied access to medical care. However, Goodin (1995) doubts that utilitarianism as a public philosophy would be committed to these unfair distributions. He argues that utilitarianism involves adopting practices and policies that are publicly accessible and long lasting. Any perverse policies, such as refusing to treat particular age groups, will become common knowledge and the harmful social effects of these perverse decisions will outweigh any benefit that could be obtained in the short term. 'That fact goes some way to ensuring that utilitarianism, practised as a public philosophy, will have few of the grievous distribution conse-quences commonly supposed' (p. 22). Nevertheless, although Goodin can provide an account of how a patently unfair distribution would not be practical, it does suggest that utilitarianism cannot rule them out in principle.

It should be apparent that the point of view which underpins a rational economic approach to health service management is an utili-tarian perspective. The health economist's method for dealing with need, discussed in the previous chapter, is a preference-satisfaction version of utilitarianism. It is possible to assess the value of meeting health care need in so far as it is an instrumental means to increasing overall utility through preference-satisfaction. However, the nature of preference-satisfaction is often left unanalysed. I have argued that accounts of utility in terms of preference-satisfaction are open to objection on the grounds of social manipulation and benign paternalism. In the absence of a thorough analysis of preference-satisfaction, it leaves a rational economic approach to management with a methodology that is solely concerned with the efficiency of distributions.

Utility and QALYs

The problems that rational economic utilitarianism has in relation to the distribution of health care can be illustrated by the example of Quality Adjusted Life Years (QALYs). The QALY appears to provide a method for answering some of the complex questions about how to determine access to health care based on need when resources are limited. It is an aggregate measure of individuals' preferences about the outcomes of a range of treatment decisions in terms of increased survival and quality of life.

The impersonality of QALYs would appear to fit well with utilitarian principles since they are geared to maximise collective preference satisfaction. Indeed, health economists who are advocates of QALYs have claimed that they could be used as a rational basis for the distribution of resources to meet health care need. By calculating a cost for each QALY gained as a result of a particular health care intervention, a cost utility league table for a range of interventions can be constructed. Such a table could be used to direct resources to the most cost-effective health care interventions. However, conceptual and practical difficulties exist in the construction of a QALY league table which mean that it is unlikely that a definitive table of cost per QALY for every health care intervention could be completed. Therefore, a QALY league table would never be a valid instrument for making decisions about allocation of health resources. However, we will examine two particular questions about QALYs that relate to principles of social justice: are QALYs equitable in terms of distribution, and are they consistent with equality in respect of basic human rights?

At first sight, QALYs would appear to support equity because every person's preference is to count for one in the aggregate calculation of utility. However, as we have seen, equality in distribution does not require an equal apportionment of social benefits, on the contrary it requires that we make allocations according to need and the differing circumstances of individuals. QALYs may be of great assistance if we are simply concerned with distributing resources on the basis of efficiency, but it is important to recognise that efficiency does not amount to distributive equality on the basis of health care need. In other words, distributing resources according to a QALY league table is efficient, but it is not necessarily fair. Second, using a QALY league table to determine priorities implies that there comes a point when it is simply not efficient in terms of utility to devote further scarce health resources to high cost, low QALY interventions. At this point, proponents of QALYs would argue that such health care interventions should no longer be supported, and a person who needed one of the proscribed interventions would be denied publicly funded treatment. One of the criticisms of the Oregon experience (Klein 1991), where just such an attempt was made to draw up a league table of interventions that could be publicly supported, was that the distinction between who had a right to treatment and who did not became arbitrary from a moral point of view.

Although utilitarians recognise a moral duty of benevolence to people who suffer misfortune, that duty only extends to those cases where meeting a need for assistance maximises overall social utility. The idea of a right to assistance, such as a right to health care, is secondary to social utility. However, some utilitarians, such as Singer (1997), argue that we have a duty to take a much more generous approach to national and international welfare than we do at present, and that substantial redistribution of resources in favour of the disadvantaged is justified in order to provide this assistance. However, the difficulty for utilitarianism remains that the obligations to improve overall welfare may infringe the rights of both the giver and receiver of aid.

Egalitarian theory

One of the main criticisms of the utilitarian treatment of social justice is that it treats human rights as a means rather than ends in themselves, and that, as a result, it cannot provide an ethical account of a *fair* society. In a fair society it should be impossible to justify sacrificing anyone's civil liberties in order to obtain economic advantage.

Nor should it be possible to sacrifice an individual's civil rights in order to increase the well-being of others, even if the others were in the majority.

John Rawls' (1971) theory of social justice is in the tradition of liberal deontological theorists who regard rights as primary and inseparable from an idea of the good. Rawls proposes that a fair society rests on two basic principles. The 'liberty principle' maintains that a fair society should maximise the civil rights of each individual. The liberty principle entails that we should strive to increase the civil liberties of all citizens, and that we help those who through no fault of their own find their liberty restricted by disease or disadvantage. The second principle, which is secondary to the liberty principle, is a 'difference principle'. This principle entails that a fair society can support economic and social differences between the most and least advantaged only in so far as the inequalities can be justified in the interests of enhancing the life prospects and benefits enjoyed by the most disadvantaged in society. It is important to note that the liberty principle and the difference principle introduce a prioritisation in distribution of benefits. First, any distribution of benefits should favour maximising liberty. Second, it should aim to favour the least advantaged within the restraints imposed by the difference principle.

These principles favour distributive equality because they require that the disadvantaged are disproportionately helped in order to obtain the same opportunities as those more favoured in life's lottery. Although this would legitimate some redistribution of social resources, Rawls proposes a limit to the redress that can be carried out in favour of the most disadvantaged. The difference principle allows that trying to even out all inequalities may prove counterproductive for the economic system, on which all depend, but which may not be able to support such a redistribution of resources. Every society depends upon healthy, productive individuals, and a balance of redistribution that does not favour this group may, in the end, worsen the conditions of the vulnerable and disadvantaged.

Rawls argues that his two principles form the basis of a social contract. The idea of the social contract is intended to demonstrate how collective political obligations and social rights rely upon the unforced consent of rational individuals. Rawls argues that his two principles of social justice can be justified through a simple thought experiment. He asks what principles of justice would rational individuals choose to underpin a fair society if they did not know beforehand their talents, interests, health or place in that society. This collective decision about social justice has be made behind a 'veil of ignorance' regarding their gender, race, intelligence, inheritance, physical characteristics and so on. Rawls argues that the liberty principle and the difference principle are those that rational people choosing the principles of social justice from behind a 'veil of ignorance' would agree on. One of the consequences of the thought experiment of choosing the principles of justice from behind the 'veil of ignorance' is that it identifies social justice with the task of counteracting the effects of chance and misfortune on people's life prospects. The 'liberty principle' would appear to support the idea that every citizen should have a 'fair opportunity' (Daniels 1985); an equal chance to participate in the benefits of society and to pursue his or her own goals, and that positive action should be taken to increase the opportunities of the least advantaged. The principle of 'fair opportunity' has clear parallels with the argument for the recognition of fundamental human needs suggested by Doyal & Gough (1991) which was introduced in the previous chapter.

A social contract based on 'fair opportunity' recognises the responsibility that we have to meet individuals' fundamental needs in order to enhance their life opportunities, and to support a health care system that attempts to prevent or ameliorate the effects of disease or injury in reducing the life opportunities open to the individual. It can be argued that such a social contract, based on the rational decisions of individuals choosing the principles of social justice from behind the 'veil of ignorance', will support some social consensus about duties of care and reciprocal positive rights to assistance. Individuals behind the veil of ignorance, unsure of their own need for health care, would agree that some health needs should be met through collective social provision. This is consistent with nurses' views about the NHS providing an implicit social consensus that legitimates the idea of a right to health care. A social contract based on Rawls' (1971) two principles of social justice can be used to justify the view that some basic health care needs should be met through state intervention. Rawls' theory of justice gives some legitimacy to claims about the duty to provide care and a positive right to have health care needs satisfied. However, it is clear that it cannot support an unlimited right to have health care needs satisfied, nor the claim that everybody's health care needs should be met by state intervention.

Entitlement theory

Rawls' theory of justice provoked trenchant criticism from libertarian philosophers who hold that a just society must protect the liberty of its citizens from interference. Nozick (1974) argues that 'patterned' theories of justice which define social justice in terms of an end state or final distribution of social benefits, such as utilitarian or egalitarian theories, will always be upset by individual liberty. People who are free to act collectively or individually in accordance with their own interests will always make choices that disrupt an ideal distribution of social benefits. Any attempt to rectify a distribution of social benefits in favour of the ideal will inevitably infringe the rights of individuals to retain their justly acquired resources, or dispose of them as they please. Nozick's entitlement theory of justice is based on a formal principle of equality that ensures that resources are justly acquired and transferred between individuals, and that just rectification is made where resources are acquired unjustly. It is argued that intervention to redress social inequalities is unfair, since it will result in the curtailment of individual liberty, and it will reduce the incentive to succeed which may be to the detriment of all. Indeed, Adam Smith, the 18th century philosopher, famously claimed that a formal principle of equality, in itself, will achieve a fair distribution of benefits:

> The rich only select from the heap what is most precious and agreeable. They consume little more than the poor, and in spite of their natural selfishness and rapacity ... They divide with the poor the produce of all their improvements. They are led by an invisible hand to make nearly the same distribution of the necessities of life which would have been made had the earth been divided into equal portions; ...
>
> (Smith 1759: from 11th edition, 1808, Vol. 1, p. 443)

A libertarian approach to social justice holds that the only fair distribution of benefits is that which is achieved through the just operation of a free market economy. A libertarian theory of justice gained a certain influence in British and American policy during the last decade, where it was held that minimal state intervention in a free market economy was not only the most efficient way of distributing resources but it was also the fairest. Some economists of the right do not believe that there is any morally desirable outcome of social policy over and above leaving it to individuals to decide for themselves (Green 1990).

In terms of health and welfare provision libertarians stress that it is up to individuals to buy the services they want for themselves and provide charity for the services they want others to have. Libertarians recognise that people have a duty to act charitably to aid those who suffer misfortune or illness. Nevertheless, they argue that there cannot be a right to *have* certain social benefits, such as health care, since it would involve an attempt to coerce people into accepting interests that are not their own. Welfare should be left to individuals in the form of charity. Beauchamp & Childress (1994) claim that libertarians, using a version of the 'invisible hand' argument, will accept that individuals' recognition of their moral duties will result in them acting generously and benevolently through voluntary rather than coercive means in order to provide an equivalent level of resources to sustain a right to health care as if it were achieved through taxation.

INDIVIDUALISM AND SOCIAL JUSTICE

One response to the controversy about the nature of social justice is to point to the apparent impossibility of ending this debate. The problem, as MacIntyre (1981, 1988) sees it, arises because all sides of the debate espouse the view that the basic moral value is the individual's pursuit of his or her own values and purposes, and that this places no limits as to what the individual can choose as his or her goal. Utilitarians acknowledge the aggregate of individual preference-satisfaction at the heart of their conception of the good. Libertarians and egalitarians base their account of rights and duties on the preservation of individual choice and autonomy. MacIntyre objects to this individualism about values because it infects moral discourse with an 'emotivist' language, moral debate is concerned with individuals' expression of their own preferences, and the use of instrumental reason and authority to persuade others to act in accordance with their wishes. The interminability of the resulting political debate arises because addressing moral questions in this way makes them insoluble in principle since there is no common moral framework for consensus. He argues that utilitarian, egalitarian and libertarian theories provide a permissive and individualistic account of social justice that defines it in terms of allowing individuals to pursue whatever goals they value. He points out that a permissive account fails to give any moral content to the idea of social justice since it separates the purpose of social justice from a common moral purpose for humanity.

In the previous chapter I argued that MacIntyre attempts to rediscover an Aristotelian notion of the *telos* of humanity, an objective account of the purpose of human life in terms of human flourishing or the pursuit of human excellence. On MacIntyre's view, ideas of human flourishing are partly determined by social and historical context and dependent upon the possibility of social participation. The moral content to the idea of social justice is given by the objective criteria by which a society encourages the pursuit of human excellence or the good life.

MacIntyre's critique of modernity and current ethical debate is compelling. However, it seems possible to argue that Rawls' (1971) theory is not an attempt to base social justice on the kind of rational individualism that MacIntyre deplores. Although Rawls' use of the 'veil of ignorance' may appear to be an attempt to use rational individualism, stripped of cultural or historical context, to provide the resources for a theory of social justice, it should be recalled that it is *only* a thought experiment to show just how far we do have a common frame of reference and a collective interest in cooperation. Rawls' account does not appear incompatible with the view that a just society is one which maintains institutions that allow the pursuit of human excellence and recognise that ideals of human excellence are essentially contestable, rather than one that imposes a particular conception of social justice on its citizens.

CONCLUSION

In the previous chapter I made a case for the idea of objective health care need, although it was accepted that such needs may be contested according to different conceptions of human harm and flourishing. In this chapter I have argued that a fair allocation of health care resources would allow a distribution of resources according to objective health care need. However, treating people fairly does not mean that everyone gets the same, and moral disagreement over whose needs should have priority is complicated by different perspectives on the seriousness of an individual's need, the visibility of that need, and the visibility of the opportunity costs in meeting it. These differences about the seriousness and visibility of need are informed by competing theories of social justice, and are complicated by a lack of consensus about the social goals of the NHS.

All theories of social justice would appear to support the notion that we have a duty to provide assistance to those in need of care. However, they differ about whether a need for health care amounts to a right to health care, and whether the State has a role in funding or providing health services to meet those needs. An egalitarian theory of social justice based on a liberty principle and a difference principle supports the notion that people ought to have a fair opportunity in life which entails some kind of reciprocal agreement that requires us to assist in the welfare of others. The NHS would seem to represent just such a recognition of our collective social responsibility to meet peoples' health care needs, and provides the basis for an implicit agreement which legitimates nurses' and health professionals' claims about the positive rights of people in need of care. On the other hand, health managers, planners and policy makers often draw upon a utilitarian language that is concerned with opportunity costs and the most efficient means to maximise utility within fixed resources without any reference to rights. Competing with these views is a libertarian perspective that emphasises the importance of negative rights; this view denies the validity of a positive right to *receive* a social benefit such as health care or the State's redistributing social resources in order to meet people's health care needs.

MacIntyre's (1988) criticism of the attempt to base principles of social justice on rational individualism identifies just how far a specifically moral conception of the purpose of social justice has become lost. Libertarians do not concern themselves with the consequences of actions on social justice. They are solely concerned with just social processes that preserve individual rights. On the other side, utilitarians are solely concerned with the consequences of actions on social utility, but where social utility has no other moral purpose than individual preference-satisfaction. However, I suggest that Rawls' (1971) version of an egalitarian theory of social justice, based on principles that promote an equal share in the success of society, can be seen as consistent with MacIntyre's teleological conception of a moral purpose for social justice. Although Rawls' thought experiment about people who have to choose the principles of social justice from behind the veil of ignorance seems to require us to consider how they would decide on the basis of their own self-interest, another way of viewing the thought experiment is to see it as an argument for mutual aid. The moral content of Rawls' theory is based on an agreement for the establishment of social institutions that ameliorate disadvantage, promote social participation, and maintain the conditions for re-evaluation of the goals of social justice.

The objective account of need presented in the previous chapter draws upon the conditions for human flourishing that can provide a basis for consensus about the necessity of meeting certain recognised needs. An egalitarian theory of social justice provides support for social institutions such as the NHS designed to meet these socially recognised needs, and justifies the redistribution of resources to do so. Although the scope, urgency and priority of these socially recognised needs will remain contested, the principles of social justice that underpin egalitarian institutions require the protection of mechanisms for debate about the relative priority and urgency of socially recognised needs. It follows that a right to health care is not fixed, and it will depend upon the scope of the consensus about socially recognised need. A right will also depend upon consensus about making the requisite health care resources available. Rawls' difference principle reminds us that excessive redistribution in favour of meeting health care needs may work to the general disadvantage of all by undermining the stability and economic viability of society.

REFERENCES

Aquinas T 1224/5–1274 Summa theologica II. In: Clark M (ed) 1972 An Aquinas reader. Fordham University Press, New York
Aristotle 384–322 BC Nichomachean ethics. In: McKeon R (ed) 1941 The basic works of Aristotle. Random House, New York
Arthur J 1997 Rights and the duty to bring aid. In: LaFollette H (ed) Ethics in practice: an anthology. Blackwell, Oxford
Beauchamp T, Childress J 1994 Principles of biomedical ethics, 4th edn. Oxford University Press, Oxford
Bentham J 1843 Anarchical fallacies. Reprinted in: Waldron J 1987 'Nonsense on stilts': Bentham, Burke and Marx on the rights of man. Methuen, London
Campbell A, Charlesworth M, Gillett G, Jones G 1997 Medical ethics, 2nd edn. Oxford University Press, Oxford
Daniels N 1985 Just health care. Cambridge University Press, New York
Doyal L, Gough I 1991 A theory of human need. Macmillan, Basingstoke
Goodin R 1995 Utilitarianism as a public philosophy. Cambridge University Press, Cambridge

Green D 1990 Introduction: a missed opportunity. In: Green D (ed) The NHS reforms: whatever happened to consumer choice? The Institute for Economic Affairs Health and Welfare Unit, London

Klein R 1991 On the Oregon trail; rationing health care. British Medical Journal 301: 1–2

Lukes S 1974 Power: a radical view. Macmillan, London

MacIntyre A 1981 After virtue, a study in moral theory. Duckworth, London

MacIntyre A 1988 Whose justice, which rationality. Duckworth, London

Nagel T 1979 Mortal questions. Cambridge University Press, Cambridge

Nozick R 1974 Anarchy, State and Utopia. Blackwell, Oxford

Rawls J 1971 A theory of justice. Oxford University Press, Oxford

Robinson J, Elkan R 1996 Health needs assessment: theory and practice. Churchill Livingstone, Edinburgh

Singer P 1997 Famine, affluence, and morality. In: LaFollette H (ed) Ethics in practice: an anthology. Blackwell, Oxford

Smith A 1808 The theory of moral sentiments, 11th edn. Bell and Bradfute; W Laing; and Mundell, Doig and Stevenson, Edinburgh, vol 1

Thompson I, Melia K, Boyd K 1994 Nursing ethics, 3rd edn. Churchill Livingstone, Edinburgh

United Kingdom Central Council for Nursing, Midwifery and Health Visiting (UKCC) 1992 Code of professional conduct. UKCC, London

Watson K 1997 Economic evaluation of health care. In: Jenkinson C (ed) Assessment and evaluation of health and medical care: a methods text. Open University Press, Buckingham

Managers and measurement: taking a literary approach to managerial discourse

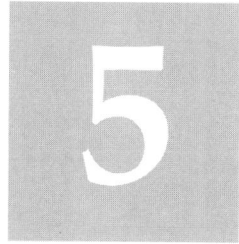

5

Michael Traynor

■ CONTENTS

Introduction   119
Recent changes to the UK
    National Health Service   120
    Strengthening central
        surveillance and control   121
    The 'internal market'   121
    Managerialism   123
    The problem with
        managerialism   123
Study design and an unexpected
    exit   124

The interviews   125
The texts   127
What has this analytical approach
    achieved?   135
    Language and power   136
    The privileging of
        measurement   137
    Measurement in the face of
        ultimate uncertainty   137
References   138

INTRODUCTION

January 31st 1989 will go down in history for two reasons. The first is that this was my last working day as an employee of the United Kingdom (UK) National Health Service (NHS). The second is that this day marked the announcement by the Thatcher Government of its ambitious plan to 'reform' the NHS involving the radical notion of the 'internal market' and the chance for the providers of NHS services to 'opt out', supposedly, of central control, that socialist anachronism. This was the latest in a series of major structural changes that angered some, excited others but probably bewildered the great majority of nurses, doctors and other clinicians working in the NHS. This chapter focuses on the words of those whose imaginations were caught by promises of a new freedom from central control, by the challenge of competition and by the chance to 'start a new culture' within the newly fashioned NHS 'trusts'. This was a period characterised by a flurry of capital investment and redecoration, where the sound of drills and hammers punctuate the optimistic aphorisms of managers captured on interview tapes, where mission statements appeared on walls, where dowdy nurse managers emerge, reconfigured in their organisation's livery, and nurses, porters and entrance halls are visually transformed for the sake of corporate ownership and local public pride.

It was also a time for old scores to be settled, with the powerful hospital consultant, and perhaps medicine in general, standing to lose the most in a contest for control over NHS resources. How far things really changed is difficult to say but there was much fighting talk, with managers, nurse managers included, offering their confrontation of medical recalcitrance as evidence of their own new potency.

RECENT CHANGES TO THE UK
NATIONAL HEALTH SERVICE

Over the previous decade and a half, UK governments at both ends of the established political spectrum, though mainly those representing the 'New Right', had brought in a range of measures aimed at controlling the activities of the large number of state-employed health professionals (Pollitt 1991). At the forefront of these groups, in the health sector, were doctors whose activities had ever-growing implications for expenditure. The Government looked to the practices of private sector organisations with their presumed efficiency to address this task. The 1980s saw the introduction of general management after the Griffiths enquiry into NHS organisation by the managing director of a leading retail chain (DHSS 1983, Paton & Bach 1990), discussed by Jane Robinson in Chapter 1, and the 1990s were to see the 'internal market' (DoH 1989, Ham 1991). In this way, 'managerialism' and market-type competition made their way into the health service, as they did into other branches of the public sector, from industry and commerce.

Involving doctors in management, for example in the clinical directorate, represented one attempt to align medicine's interests to the overall management agenda of the NHS by making them take responsibility for the financial implications of their clinical decisions. However, many doctors who took up this invitation were dismayed to find how unpopular they became with their colleagues (Drife &

Johnston 1995). The nurse executive position on the boards of the new trusts can perhaps be understood in a similar light, exchanging this alignment of interests for a sense of new participation in health service management. Indeed, the NHS Executive document, *One year On: the nurse executive director post* (NHSME 1992) presents as a key achievement that nurses have been taken seriously as managers. Indeed, with so much to prove, and with the language of corporatism as against the tribalism of the professionals achieving such dominance, it is hard to imagine how nurse executives could find it easy to be champions of nursing and represent nursing interests.

Strengthening central surveillance and control

The NHS reforms to be discussed in this and the next chapter, were brought about through the NHS and Community Care Act 1990. The scheme was set out in the White Paper *Working for Patients* (DoH 1989). District and regional health authorities were reconstituted as boards with executive and non-executive directors, the latter appointed by government ministers or regions. One commentator suggested that:

> The NHS acquired a management culture of command and obedience more usually associated with private businesses than with public services in which those who failed to toe the policy line could be penalised in their career advancements and those who criticised it could place themselves at risk of disciplinary action.
>
> (Butler 1992, p. 36)

The policy of centralising control over decision-making while decentralising activity reflected a general trend in industry, a trend facilitated by the rise of information technology (IT) with its ability (in theory at least) to monitor from the centre performance at the periphery (Klein 1989). Pollitt described the increased possibility for detailed day-to-day surveillance facilitated by this rise in IT as 'the information Panopticon' (Pollitt 1993, p. 117).

The 'internal market'

The 1991 reforms, most notably, set up the 'internal market' in state health care. The key premise of *Working for Patients* (DoH 1989) was that if health care institutions were made to compete against each other this would result not only in greater efficiency but in improved responsiveness to its consumers (Harrison et al 1990). One of the originators of the plan was American, Alain Enthoven (1985).

It brought the separation of the *provision* of services from their *purchase*, or commission (the allocation of funds for provision to meet local population health needs). Institutions were able to apply to the Secretary of State to become self-governing 'NHS Trusts'.

The advantages for trusts of this independence included freedom from nationally agreed conditions of service for their employees and greater freedom in managing their own finances with the ability to borrow capital and accumulate surpluses for reinvestment. 57 trusts were established in 1991 and 113 applications were made for the 1992 second wave of which 99 were successful (Wistow 1992). By April 1993, there were 330 trusts (Bartlett & Le Grand 1994). In April 1994, the last year of the study, 143 hospitals and community units became trusts making the total 419 representing 96% of hospital and community services (Health Service Journal 1994).

In primary care, general practitioners (GPs) with over 9000 (7000 from April 1993) patients were given the opportunity to become 'fundholders'. Fundholders received a budget from the Regional Health Authority (RHA), which, in addition to contributions towards prescribing and staff salaries received by all GPs, contained an amount reflecting the practice's potential hospital referrals for certain procedures, based, initially, on its pre-application spending level. Corresponding amounts were deducted from the allocations of strategic authorities, i.e. District Health Authorities (DHAs). The commissioning responsibility of DHAs would thus steadily diminish as the number of fundholders increased (Butler 1992). First-wave GP fundholders came into existence on 1 April 1991 and in that year were awarded a special £16 000 start-up grant as well as a £33 000 annual management fee (Holliday 1992). In April 1993, the scheme was extended. Fundholding GPs were given budgets to purchase district nursing and health visiting services from NHS community units. The guidance expressly excluded the direct employment of community nurses. In April 1994, a further 850 GP practices joined the fundholding scheme so that, at that time, 36% of the population were on the lists of such practices (Health Service Journal 1994). A further extension of the fundholding scheme took place in 1994 enabling a wider range of GPs to join the scheme, and further changes enabled 'single-handed' GPs to participate and extend fundholding to other areas of the budget (Pollitt 1993). Thus, by the end of the study, the GP fundholding scheme was still expanding.

Managerialism

Earlier, I used the term 'managerialism'. The following quotation suggests a useful summary of a managerialist world view:

> the world should be a place where objectives are clear, where staff are highly motivated to achieve them, where close attention is given to monetary costs, where bureaucracy and red tape are eliminated. If one asks how this is to be achieved the managerialist answer is, overwhelmingly, through the introduction of good management practices, which are assumed to be found at the highest pitch and most widely distributed in the private sector.
>
> (Pollitt 1993, p. 7)

Some of the roots of managerialism can be located in the 'scientific management' promoted by Frederick Winnslow Taylor, an American industrialist writing at the beginning of this century. His belief was that 'the whole country [was] suffering through inefficiency'. The remedy lay in 'systematic management' which was 'a true science, resting upon clearly defined laws, rules and principles, as a foundation' (Taylor 1911). His principles involved observation and measurement of output and the introduction of specific modifications such as rewards aimed at increasing worker performance. Since Taylor's ideas, however, successive sophistications, many associated with the influence of industrial psychologists, have involved deeper penetrations into the consciousness of the worker and attempts to place him or her at the disposal of the manager's objectives (Pollitt 1993, p. 7).

The problem with managerialism

In this chapter and the next I plan to examine issues of persuasion and manipulation as they are effected through language. The issue of manipulation and the 'redescription' (Ricoeur 1986, p. 22) of reality through rhetoric is apparent in the attention to organisational culture that gained ascendancy in managerial literature during the 1980s and early 1990s and which, perhaps in the last decade, entered NHS managerial discourse (Pollitt 1991).

While not supplanting the continuing emphasis on economy and efficiency, this new drive adds to it notions such as 'cultural change'. The successful marketing of notions such as that of 'organisational culture', and the advantages to managers of an awareness of this phenomenon have spread its popularity into the public sector. Popular management writers such as Peters and Waterman advocate attention to this aspect of organisational life and a host of others emphasise the crucial importance of the manager's initial target for change being the ideas of the workforce rather than its roles and structures (Spurgeon & Barwell 1991, Van de Ven 1980). The ultimate end, however, is instrumental, that is, increased organisational performance or increased market share or commercial survival, and its chief assumption is that those who run the organisation are the most appropriate people to determine the organisation's culture. In the present study, one manager explicitly, and almost every other manager implicitly paid allegiance to these notions. The creed of managerialism holds deep dangers. In the following quotation, the location of managerialism within both a growing social movement and a distinctively modern project is beginning to be made clear:

> Efficiency, speed, precise measurement, rationality, productivity, and technical improvement become ends in themselves, applied obsessively to areas in life in which they would previously have been rejected as inappropriate. Efficiency – the quest for maximum output per unit – is, no one would question, of paramount importance in technical systems. But now efficiency takes on a more general value and becomes a universal maxim for all intelligent conduct.
>
> (Winner 1977)

The mantle of neutrality

Philosopher Alistair MacIntyre sees 'the manager' as one of the three central characters on the contemporary social stage (MacIntyre 1985). He critiques managers' claims to effectiveness and neutrality by arguing that such claims to effectiveness are morally implicated because they are 'inseparable from a mode of human existence in which the contrivance of means is in central part the manipulation of human beings into compliant patterns of behaviour' (MacIntyre 1985, p. 74).

It is managerial rhetorical practice, coupled with claims to rationality, cloaked with the 'mantle of neutrality' that I would like to focus on in the rest of this chapter.

STUDY DESIGN AND AN UNEXPECTED EXIT

This chapter and the next arise from my work at the Daphne Heald Research Unit at the Royal College of Nursing in the UK. The research initially took place in the first four first-wave NHS community-based trusts to agree to participate, and proceeded over 4 years. Although essentially a convenience sample because of the need to start the study as quickly as possible after the reforms were implemented, the trusts differed in organisational structure and in the type of locality within which they operated. However, these factors appeared to have little influence on the managerial discourses and rhetoric adopted. The management of one of the trusts withdrew from the study after receiving the report of the first year's findings for that trust. The findings indicated low morale among the workforce and a great many extremely critical comments about management – a similar picture to the other trusts. (The workforce in this organisation did indeed have the lowest job satisfaction in the study.) The management team of this trust were only too aware of these problems, but solving them did not involve further participation in a study which they saw as partisan and with an undeclared 'trust-bashing' agenda.

A summary of the management interviews carried out is given in Table 5.1. The trust that withdrew, Trust 2, is excluded from the table and from discussion. Trust 1a represents an attempt to include in the study the health visiting service in that part of the country which was located, not in the community trust (Trust 1), but in the acute trust. The first year interviews took place between April and September, 1992; the second year between May and September, 1993; and the final year interviews between March and October, 1994.

The interviews

The interviews lasted an average of 50 minutes, were tape recorded and transcribed in full. The questions addressed were extremely wide-ranging.

I focused attention upon 19 interviews in order to undertake close textual analysis. They comprise interviews carried out with nine individuals and one small group interview with a team of three managers of health visitors, making a total of 12 individuals. Two of this sample of 12 managers were men. The individuals were; three nurse executives, three chief executives and one senior community manager from the trust where community nurses were managed in a separate directorate. These texts were chosen because they were produced from interviews with individuals in leading positions in their organisations. They were likely to present the 'official' views of the organisation. In addition certain interviews with managers who expressed clearly sceptical views about the reforms and certain aspects of their organisations were also selected for close analysis. These were a nurse adviser and a locality manager from one of the

Table 5.1 Table of interviews: all years

Trust	Year		
	1	2	3
Trust 1			
Chief Executive	X		X
Nurse Executive	X	X	X
Nurse Adviser	X		
Locality Manager 1	X		X
Locality Manager 2	X		X
Locality Manager 3	X		
Locality Manager 4	X		X
Trust 1a			
Two senior managers of the health visiting service together (three in year 3)	X	X	X
Trust 3			
Chief Executive	X		X
Nurse Executive	X		X
Director Primary Care	X		X
Assistant Director Primary Care	X		X
Locality Manager 1	X	X	X
Locality Manager 2	X		X
Locality Manager 3	X	X	X
Locality Manager 4	X		X
Trust 4			
Chief Executive	X		X
Nurse Executive	X	X	X
Director of Local Services	X		X
Nurse Adviser	X	X	X
Locality Manager 1	X		
Locality Manager 2	X		
Neighbourhood Manager 1	X		X
Neighbourhood Manager 2	X		
Neighbourhood Manager 3			X
Neighbourhood Manager 4			X

trusts and the small management team of three health visitors from another trust. Analysis of the sample of 19 interviews was greatly helped by the use of the computer program, NUD*IST v.3.0 (Richards & Richards 1994). A range of differences that were expected at the out-set of the research between the discourse of, for example, executives with nursing and those with administrative backgrounds, between the male and female managers and between the different years of the study were hard to detect with any confidence.

It became clear, particularly as I explored the literature mentioned in the introduction to the book, that the analysis of the interviews and questionnaire comments could be taken in an entirely different direction to that of the original purposes of the research. Rather than concentrate on the 'factual answers' to the questions, or on the intentional 'meaning' of those interviewed, I sensed that an analysis of the language that flowed through their arguments, almost as if it had an independent existence of its own, might provide some knowledge of the discourses at work in contemporary UK health care.

The texts

The next section of this chapter gives examples of explorations of notions of the rationality of measurement and of financial constraint.

Measurement

There is detectable in the interviews a sense in which knowledge was not trustworthy or legitimate unless it took a particular form that we might describe as measurement. To know what nurses were doing, to describe the organisation, the basis of interactions between organisations all required measurement of increasing sophistication. The metaphors most often associated with understanding were visual; 'we are looking at ...' As knowledge became more synonymous with information stored electronically as a series of zeros and ones, measurement became the symbol of objectivity, of a metaphysical pursuit of the original, the trustworthy, the real. Numerical information represented the rejection of language-dependent knowledge and subjectivity. Yet no matter how strenuously this abstraction was sought, subjective and interested decisions about what activities to record, how they might be represented, what forces were allowed to remain invisible, financial pressures and incentives, 'visions', grudges and beliefs all haunted the margins of their exclusion. The encounter between reason and ignorance staged at times by the managers dissolves into a much more evenly matched contest as the interviews demonstrated not so much the managers' command of verifiable information as their great skill at the art of rhetoric.

Whether they liked it or not, managers were at the centre of political attention, having committed themselves to the Government's reforms. Although many involved in this research hinted that their own personal politics were far from those of the Thatcher administration, they had taken up its call for 'more efficient' public sector management. This decision having been taken, they were then already in a position of having to defend a particular range of interests against those of other groups who did not identify with the Government or its NHS reforms and who attacked them.

For example, in the early days of the reforms, rumour and incomplete knowledge appeared to abound within the organisations under study. Some managers believed much of this to be political in nature. This was excluded as invalid, subjective knowledge. One way to counter its influence was with the 'facts'; perhaps the Chief Executive would carry out a 'lecture tour' of staff bases to counteract these forces with some hard data. The aim might be to:

> tell people [staff] how we are doing, how we did last year, how many patients we saw, how that was better than the year before, what our financial position was at the end of the year, so that people actually know how the trust did, so it's first hand, rather than sort of a jaded documentary on Channel Four.
>
> (Trust 1 Nurse Executive)

In this passage reliable knowledge is contrasted with another type of knowledge, a 'jaded documentary on Channel Four'. A television 'documentary' might carry connotations of factual reportage and insight so the addition of 'jaded' acts as an adjective to discredit this reading. The words 'sort of' alert us that the speaker is searching, perhaps with studied carelessness but with much cynicism, for an exemplar of a biased media report so that it is clear that the 'jaded documentary' in question could either be a stereotype or an actual program. For the purposes of his discrediting act it does not matter which. 'Channel Four' adds to the effect. The UK's avowedly unconventional and radical television channel can be easily marginalised as biased and non-serious. The purportedly political motivation of the media report is contrasted with supposedly value-free knowledge of numerical measurement of balance sheets, 'our financial position', 'how many patients we saw' and trends of increasing throughput, like the soaring lines on graphs seen on the walls of the Trust Chair's offices during this research. These are described as the verifiable facts of the situation.

Managers were keen that nurses should learn that it was in their interests to take up the same approach to knowledge so that their claims, for example about staffing inadequacies, might be taken as legitimate rather than seen as the gendered workplace equivalent of nagging. This would involve learning to speak and think more numerically and in more detailed a fashion about the 'information' on 'patient dependency'. Valid knowledge is therefore disembodied knowledge, a numerical account:

> I met the Day Ward Sister on my rounds and she was *on about staffing* and I said 'you have evidence here of that' and she'd done no record of patient dependency.
>
> (Trust 3 Nurse Executive – my emphasis)

Mechanisms were created for the detailed and constant measurement and recording of a particular kind of information. (These were the systems for monitoring nursing activity, the introduction of which Jane Robinson refers to in Chapter 1. Here, more than half a decade later, they have been extended so that every nurse is expected to be aware of their relevance and utility.) Again the emphasis is on quantities, levels, numerical patterns, disembodied knowledge:

> what we are doing is monitoring very carefully the referral rate to our community nursing team. We did an awful lot of benchmark work prior to April 1st so that referral patterns, trends, volume we knew, the number of people who we were supporting in residential homes we knew so that we could pick up any increases, any trends.
>
> (Trust 1 Nurse Executive)

Managers were frank about the limitations of their knowledge of nursing work, yet computer-based activity remained the 'foundation' for knowledge and the most reliable way of grasping and describing so-called 'quality' of care:

> We've spent a lot of money … developing an information system that will collect information and we're really still at the stage of trying to implement that community system, which is the foundation to actually being able to report on quality outcomes and until that's in place it's going to be quite difficult to get any meaningful information.
>
> (Trust 1 Chief Executive)

There is an appeal to a technological discourse that associates notions of dependability, authority and thoroughness with computers: 'We've spent a lot of money developing' a 'system'. Talk about 'quality' has become here methodical and impersonal yet reliable and trustworthy because of these very qualities; an 'information system' that appears to 'collect' its own 'information'. Understanding the quality of care is described in a way that equates, or at least associates, it with computer activity, to 'report on quality outcomes'. The language is free from any suggestion of subjectivity or value which within this discourse would undermine the authority of the 'foundation'. Both are present, though erased from the discourse, in the very design of 'the system', of what constitutes 'information' and what 'information' to request. Information is never simply collected. Yet, in spite of this foundation of impersonality, there is, perhaps paradoxically, meaning to be found; 'meaningful information'. Managers often expressed a preference for formalised, numerically based information over and above knowledge gained through 'going out with the nurses personally' and 'being told by the nurses' even though the former was acknowledged as sometimes grossly inaccurate. This preference is supported by appeals to scientific discourse evident in terms such as 'measure' and 'indicator' with connotations of objectivity. These analytical tools are associated in the following passage, which deals with changing workload levels, with metaphors of penetration and deep knowledge, a dualistic getting beyond the appearances to the reality of the situation. 'Meaning' is excluded rhetorically, chased off limits, in the language with which knowledge and measurement is described, yet it haunts the managerial discourse:

> people might say that's an incredibly crude measure, it nevertheless is one measure we can use in terms of did it take two nurses an hour and a half to deal with someone rather than one nurse 10 minutes and you know that gives you some basic indicators to help you delve into the issues.
>
> (Trust 4 Nurse Executive)

In keeping with an emphasis on measurement and measurability, relationships between health care organisations tended to be numerically based, with formal verifiable agreements, the contracting at the heart of the reforms. For example service agreements might mean that every GP will 'know exactly what input he's going to get' (Trust 1 Chief Executive) where the mechanistic 'input' means the number of hours worked, by nurses graded at particular levels of skill. The regular and timely completion of generalised and abstracted 'activity' recording on the part of staff is a vital first link in the contractual process and bears a direct relation to financial income for the trust:

> Now, we're monitoring on a month-by-month basis and I get my information on monthly activity in 10 days from the end of the month and we have an agreement with – a contract with the Commission that as

soon as I identify a real increase in activity, then we will sit down and renegotiate the contract.

(Trust 1 Nurse Executive)

Contractual agreements did not always appear to be purely numerically based, yet the repetition of 'evidence' in the reading from the 'quality' document below and the description of the 'monitoring' and 'reports that ... demonstrate' lead quickly into numerically presented 'evidence'. The language is intentionally of binary certainty, either the criteria have been met or they have not:

Evidence that staff resources are targeted in areas where there is a high risk in child protection work; evidence that health service staff have been offered the correct immunisation by the occupational health department; evidence of appropriate staff update in current techniques and emergency procedures ... and what we do in our monitoring meeting is we provide reports that will demonstrate, for example, the numbers of areas of training, how many staff have been trained and in which specific areas ....

(Trust 3 Community Manager)

Only one nurse executive offered a detailed response to the problem of the quantifiability of nursing work. However, her politically pragmatic solution amounted to the recommendation that it was in nurses' interests to adopt the dominant language and mentality of numerical measurement even though she distances herself from it at the beginning of the passage. She effects this by ascribing it to 'men in the medical profession' and referring to measurement as if it were a meaningless or automatic activity 'the numbers game' and 'number crunching':

One of the things that happens in health care is that if you do all the stuff that is quantifiable, like the numbers game and number crunching then you definitely can prove something in the view, I have to say it, of men in the medical profession, who think they own science and research, not all of them, but some of them ...

Her response can be understood as a struggle between an organisationally dominant discourse of measurability and demonstrability on the one hand and of the 'art' or unquantifiability of nursing work on the other. There are echoes of nursing's epistemological and political struggle with medicine which has often been identified with 'science' by nurses. The result is an ambiguous text, an example, perhaps, of postmodernism's fragmented self attempting to take a position within these two discourses simultaneously. The following passage, which occurs immediately after the previous one, can be read as an expression of the speaker's own 'dilemma':

> and I think it actually puts nurses in a very difficult dilemma, when they are coming from a very different worldview of events. … Immunisation is a classic one, it is a real number crunchy one which health visitors can get into. In a way they almost don't like doing it, they don't want, I think health visitors have got to make up their minds what it is they want to do … the trouble is that health care is so incredibly complex.

Having summarised a measurement discourse and opposed it with a description of the position of certain health care workers, the speaker goes on to offer a resolution:

> I think every nurse in the community, whoever they may be, if you are a district nurse you can measure a wound and you can measure if it is closing up or not and healing, and that is something very quantifiable. Immunisation for health visitors, I'm trying to think of something for school nursing, number of children that have less days of absenteeism from school perhaps, because they have actually dealt with the problem that was affecting their school attendance, there is all sorts of things they can use, less pregnancies …
>
> (Trust 4 Nurse Executive)

However, in the process of grasping for these examples, the character of the work done by these nurses and health visitors suffers the very reduction or erasure that the speaker has been attempting to avoid in her acknowledgement of the 'incredible complex[ity]' of health care.

As well as admitting that existing computerised systems did not at present capture enough detail of workforce activity, whether through incompleteness or lack of sophistication, managers spoke about another more fundamental kind of limitation to formal measurement. This did not, however, appear to significantly shake their faith in the centrality of such an approach in the steering of their organisations. In one significant passage, a manager completely undermines the whole foundation of measurement-based contracting by suggesting that even this apparently objective approach could be arbitrary and open to manipulation:

> The current method of face-to-face contact is not a good method. There is no quality aspect to it and you can actually manufacture face-to-face contacts to – we could almost say to the Commission, 'How many do you want us to make?' and we will make that. That's not a problem.
>
> (Trust 1 Nurse Executive)

Financial rationality

In some senses monitoring and measurement existed to underpin financial work. However, as I have hinted before, in other ways, the project of surveillance and rational control and organisation has other roots and more far-reaching effects.

Passages dealing with such forces can be separated into those in which finance was appealed to as a foundational reality from which judgements and evaluations stemmed and those which made such a point but also occurred near to passages discussing wider aspects of rationality. In this way a link was made between financial rationality and rational behaviour more broadly. Very occasionally, speakers would appear to distance themselves from a financial basis of evaluation:

> It is our intention for this trust to be successful and success means financially viable and that's a measure that's applied to us rather than one we would necessarily apply ourselves.
> [In the] 3 years leading up to becoming a trust … [we] had to become increasingly financially orientated because we were in a mess, a million and a half pounds overspent.
>
> (Trust 1 Nurse Executive)

Often, however, managers presented themselves as skilled financially, drawing power from wielding financial decision-making:

> There are huge agendas around like … for example, which mean that we are looking to try and re-provide facilities in more appropriate accommodation and all that that means, so that in the hope that new provision will be more cost-effective in the way it's delivered which will give us resources to spend on new developments, rather than continuing to provide uneconomic services.
>
> (Trust 1 Chief Executive)

> I was saving money and I said to them [district nurses] if I save money, you can have it back. So, for example, pagers, a lot of them have pagers now and that was simply because I saved money from going from a G to an E and if I save £2–3000, or whatever it was, perhaps increase a bit of bank nursing capacity, I bought pagers for everybody.
>
> (Trust 1 Nurse Executive)

Most managers welcomed, or at least adopted the rhetoric of welcoming, the financial directness of so-called market forces as reinforcing the service ethos of the NHS. In the following quotation, there is a rhetorically effected reversal, an unusual identification between the moral rhetoric of 'respect', 'dignity' and 'positive attitude' and the mechanistic 'winding down' of staffing levels. Staff should realise that it is in their interests to overcome their reluctance to deliver a caring service. It is their apparent unwillingness that is painted as a doubtful moral unknown in this situation. Market forces lend management a new authority over people – if *they* (the 'staff') fail to perform adequately *we* will respond:

> our staff will have to come to terms with it more and more. If they don't treat the purchaser and his patients with respect, with dignity, with positive attitude, they'll lose business and we'll wind down the number of staff.
>
> (Trust 3 Chief Executive)

Managers were able to take up a posture of neutrality by ascribing to market and financial forces a certain impersonality, an erasure of the political context of decision-making, as if 'the market', like the science of measurement or the laws of physics, has its own autonomous workings. Yet, at the same time as celebrating the disembodied existence of these forces, managers assert their own potency, as if they are acting with the flow of Nature, of an inner logic:

> what we did with the doctors last year was, they were, almost had, well, they had no job to do … It was just, the fact that GPs had taken over child surveillance, rightly or wrongly, I'm not there to comment on the politics of it, whether it's a good idea. It had happened and they just were not fully occupied so we made them redundant and I've done the same thing with the dentists last week. I made six dentists redundant.
>
> (Trust 4 Nurse Executive)

Appealing to finance as a given quantity enabled managers to adopt a rhetoric of offering freedom of choice to field staff, while actually exercising detailed control:

> I should be able to say to the nurses you have this amount of money, and I don't mind how you use it, as long as you follow these types of criteria, focus on these priorities and we expect this quality of work and we expect these hours covered.
>
> (Trust 4 Chief Executive)

In another passage, the use of language suggests that decision-making and power are exercised at the level of the individual client and health care worker. This is achieved by an appeal to notions of consumer empowerment and professional autonomy ('managing the care') and an erasing of the fact that financial decisions have already been made by a chain of politicians and bureaucrats. This last act of rhetoric is effected through the use of the highly colloquial and metaphorical 'bottom line' and 'money in the pot' suggesting commonplace and unalterable realities:

> The bottom line is that there is only so much money in the pot so they [health visitors] and the client have to decide together the best way of managing their care.
>
> (Trust 4 Nurse Executive)

WHAT HAS THIS ANALYTICAL
APPROACH ACHIEVED?

Most notably, this approach has shown how managers employ a range of rhetorical skills to further their viewpoint and marginalise those who do not share this view, while at the same time presenting themselves as rational and acting along with objective criteria. This move echoes the Socratic strategy critiqued by Derrida with its stress on the virtues of clear-cut logical analysis but its fundamental 'will to persuade' and to 'monopolise for itself all claims to reason, dignity and truth' (Norris 1991, p. 60). This research has discovered the managers as 'wily rhetorician[s]' (Norris 1991, p. 61). Ricoeur reminds us that metaphor 'redescribes' reality (Ricoeur 1986, p. 22) and that skill at rhetoric has been seen as affording its user formidable power to 'manipulate words apart from things, and to manipulate men by manipulating words' (Ricoeur 1986, p. 11). Organisational writers urge managers to accumulate such skills, although they generally erase the moral and political from their exhortations. Gahmberg describes 'metaphor management' as part of the successful manager's 'creation of a meaningful context for the organisational members' (Gahmberg 1990). Swales & Rogers argue that management literature has consistently recognised the importance of language in business affairs, that among tangible signs of change in an organisation a key one is that its language is changing; through it 'meaning is created and action becomes possible' (Swales & Rogers 1995, p. 224). I would suggest that the texts analysed in this chapter offer examples of just such attempts at the creation of meaning.

MacIntyre addresses the notion of manipulation when considering the managerial claim to moral neutrality and to its own effectiveness, which he considers central to the way that contemporary managers present themselves. He first demonstrates that anyone wishing to persuade another to carry out a particular course of action has two different approaches at his or her disposal. The first is the use of personal criteria where the hearer's decision to act depends upon a range of personal and contextual factors 'do this because I wish it'. The second, which MacIntyre argues is characteristic of our culture and times, involves the speaker's appeal to purportedly impersonal, rational criteria, 'do this because it is your duty' or 'do this because it would give pleasure to a number of people' or in the present case, 'do this because it is the best use of our organisation's limited funds'. The second form of persuasion can be considered manipulative persuasion because, in an age where there are no agreed and unassailable criteria for moral action, such appeals confer an objectivity on utterances that are no more than expressions of their speaker's own preference (MacIntyre 1985, p. 17).

Language and power

An analysis of language can make explicit how its use is implicated in power relationships by showing how a discourse that is dominant in a society at a particular time can be used by (and uses) those making claims for knowledge and authority. In turn, those with authority influence the culture of organisations by shaping what it is legitimate to discuss and record and therefore what has existence and what has not. For example, western society, perhaps since the Enlightenment, has taken up the challenge of emancipation from the authority of law and tradition through the use of reason. In a sense, health service managers' moves to replace the individualistic, subjective response to health care spoken of by many front-line caregivers (see the next chapter) with measurable, rationally planned activities can be seen as part of this 'modern' project.

Weber saw modern bureaucracies as mechanisms and embodiments of impersonality, impartiality and functionality in contrast – and such definitions are always dependent upon some act of exclusion – to relationships based on individual privileges and bestowal of favour which were said to characterise traditional structures (Weber 1947). 'Above all there is a separation of the public world of rationality and efficiency from the private sphere of emotional and personal life' (Pringle 1988, p.86). The managers in this study spoke about their approach in a way that often contrasted aspects of rationality with a previous or more primitive state that they encountered within their organisations. The traditional society that the managers came to reform was manifest in the ancient and arcane secrets at the heart of the Professions, knowledge that afforded professionals a privilege almost anachronistic in an age of reason. Paradoxically, medicine and, during particular stages in its history, nursing, have presented themselves in the same light, as bearers of the rationality of science. Yet a subsequent wave of rationality, taking as its point of reference financial control, has overtaken them and made them seem almost superstitious by contrast. The second tradition was of fear, ignorance and superstition embodied and traditionally associated with the womanly arts (Jordanova 1989), one of whose descendants in the modern world is the occupation of nursing. The third tradition is also associated with women; that of the realm of emotions and of the home, the site and crucible of so much emotional work. All these traditions, are pushed to the margins and excluded by a new language of rationality and measurement.

The privileging of measurement

My analysis has shown how the metaphors used by managers reinforce and extend the privilege they give to techniques of measurement by associating them with notions of penetrating appearances to reveal reality. This, along with metaphors of physical distance and mental activity help to locate their picture of knowledge within a dualism that systematically downgrades the 'embodied' knowledge claimed by front-line caregivers in their own texts.

Measurability and the development of computerised and other methods of recording and regulating activity can be seen in the light of Foucault's descriptions of the art of ever more penetrating surveillance that he argues has been a characteristic of modern European disciplinary societies (Foucault 1977). Although they exceed the specific historical contingency, these characteristics (measurement and control) are also highly compatible with government moves to contain health care spending and indeed, the whole move to measurement seems underpinned by the contracting process with its financial incentives and penalties.

Measurement in the face of ultimate uncertainty

In western health care we are faced with an ever increasing range of possible interventions and with attempts to reduce expenditure but we are faced at the same time with the loss of faith in an overarching medical authority. There are now a multiplicity of voices competing for a say on ever more complex health care decisions. The strategy of governments has lain in being seen to be making decisions on the basis of some form of rational criteria. (This need explains some of the attractiveness to government and purchasers alike of the NHS research and development strategy (DoH 1991).) '[O]bjectivist discourses are not just the territory of intellectuals and academics,' notes Sandra Harding, 'they are the official dogma of the age' (Harding 1990, p. 88). The health needs assessment that, in theory, forms the basis of the purchasing that is intended to drive the UK internal market (Ham 1991) is one such attempt. The Oregon experiment in the USA (Klevit et al 1991), in which the local population were given an opportunity to contribute to decisions about which health care procedures were funded, produced a troubling outcome, which involved vetoing of the scheme by President George Bush in 1992 (McBride 1992). In the absence of a more convincing moral consensus, the form of rationality adopted by governments has been utilitarian. If managers at the local level can direct their efforts towards the measurement, control and efficient distribution of health care inputs, they might maintain something close to the masquerade of potency that MacIntyre argues masks a fundamental powerlessness within corporations and governments (MacIntyre 1985, p. 75).

In the next chapter, I will present the highly contrasting style of the nurses' contribution to this research.

REFERENCES

Bartlett W, Le Grand J 1994 The performance of trusts. In: Robinson R, Le Grand J (eds) Evaluating the NHS reforms. King's Fund Institute, London, pp 54–73
Butler J 1992 Patients, policies and politics: before and after 'Working for patients'. Open University Press, Milton Keynes
Department of Health (DoH) 1989 Working for patients. Cmd. 555 HMSO, London
Department of Health (DoH) 1991 Research for health; a research and development strategy for the NHS. HMSO, London
Department of Health and Social Security (DHSS) 1983 NHS management inquiry report. (The Griffiths Report) DA(83)38, DHSS, London
Drife J, Johnston I 1995 Management for doctors: handling the conflicting cultures in the NHS. British Medical Journal 310(6986): 1054–1056
Enthoven A C 1985 Reflections on the management of the National Health Service: an American looks at incentives to efficiency in health services management in the UK. Nuffield Provincial Hospital Trust, London
Foucault M 1977 Discipline and punish. Penguin, Harmondsworth
Gahmberg H 1990 Metaphor management: on the semiotics of strategic leadership. In: Turner B (ed) Organizational symbolism. Walter de Gruyter, Berlin
Ham C 1991 The new national health service; organisation and management. Radcliffe Medical Press, Oxford
Harding S 1990 Feminism, science and the anti-enlightenment critiques. In: Nicholson L (ed) Feminism/postmodernism. Routledge, London, 83–106
Harrison S, Hunter D, Pollitt C 1990 The dynamics of British health policy. Unwin Hyman, London
Health Service Journal 1994 News. In brief. Health Service Journal 104(7 April): 4
Holliday I 1992 The NHS transformed. Baseline Books, Manchester
Jordanova L 1989 Sexual visions. Images of gender in science and medicine between the eighteenth and twentieth centuries. Harvester Wheatsheaf, Hemel Hempstead
Klein R 1989 The politics of the National Health Service. Longman, London

Klevit H, Bates A, Castanares T, Kirk P, Sipes-Metzler P, Wopat, R 1991 Prioritization of health care services. A progress report by the Oregon Health Services Commission. Archives of International Medicine 151(May): 912–916

MacIntyre A 1985 After virtue. A study in moral theory. Duckworth, London

McBride G 1992 Bush vetoes health care rationing in Oregon. British Medical Journal 305(22 Aug): 437

NHS and Community Care Act 1990 HMSO, London

National Health Service Management Executive (NHSME) 1992 One year on: the nurse executive director post. Report on the role and function of the nurse executive director post in first wave NHS trusts. Department of Health and Central Office of Information, London

Norris C 1991 Deconstruction; theory and practice. Routledge, London

Paton C, Bach S 1990 Case studies in health policy and management. Nuffield Provincial Hospitals Trust, London

Pollitt C 1991 The politics of quality: managers, professionals and consumers in the public services. Revised version of a public lecture. Royal Holloway and Bedford New College, Centre for Political Studies, London

Pollitt C 1993 Managerialism and the public services. Blackwell, Oxford

Pringle R 1988 Secretaries talk. Sexuality, power and work. Unwin, London

Richards T, Richards L 1994 Non-numerical unstructured data indexing, searching and theorising (NUD*IST). Qualitative Solutions and Research, Melbourne

Ricoeur P 1986 The rule of metaphor. Multi-disciplinary studies of the creation of meaning in language. Routledge, London

Spurgeon P, Barwell F 1991 Implementing change in the NHS. A guide for general managers. Chapman and Hall, London

Swales J, Rogers P 1995 Discourse and the projection of corporate culture: the Mission Statement. Discourse and Society 6(2): 223–242

Taylor F W 1911 The principles of scientific management. Harper and Brothers, New York

Van de Ven A 1980 Problem solving, planning and innovation, Part 1: Test of programme planning method; Part 2: Speculations for theory and practice. Human Relations Journal 33(Nov–Dec): 10–11

Weber M 1947 The theory of social and economic organisation. Free Press, Glencoe Ill

Winner L 1977 Autonomous technology. MIT Press, Boston

Wistow G 1992 The National Health Service. In: Marsh D, Rhodes R (eds) Implementing Thatcherite policies: an audit of an era. Open University Press, Milton Keynes, pp. 100–116

Morality and self-sacrifice in nursing talk

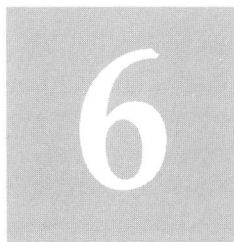

Michael Traynor

6

■ CONTENTS

Introduction 141
  Nursing as a moral activity 142
  Nursing and managerialism 145
  Introduction to the analytical
    approach: a focus on text 146
  Structuralism, semiotics
    and the 'turn to
    language' 146
  Structuralism, poststructuralism 148

Discourse analyses 149
The Royal College of Nursing
  research 150
The nurses' comments 151
The questionnaire comments:
  how nurses talked about
  their work 151
References 160

INTRODUCTION

In this chapter I would like discuss a very different range of discourses which are discernible in the comments of the nurses involved in the research which I introduced in the previous chapter. But first a word of caution.

It would be all too beguiling to oppose the arguments of the nurses and managers in the same dualistic terms in which they take each other's arguments and use them for their own projects. The success of the managers' project depends, in part, upon how well they can present clinicians as irrational, self-seeking, financially profligate and, hence, in need of control. Clinicians, for their part, have sought public support by pointing to the contradiction between managers' talk of efficiency and their expansion in numbers and cost, or by characterising them as spiritual philistines, tainted and limited by their association with industry and commerce, excluded from the intimacy, humanity – and power – of the clinician's relationship with the patient. However, the power and effect of the dualism that both groups draw upon depends on ambient cultural dualisms, between rationality and irrationality, for example. If I use the same dualisms that the actors in this research do, I argue that while it is beyond our hopes to sweep these dualisms away, we can destabilise them. We can show, in this instance, how two groups depend on them to further their own projects even relying upon some vital aspect of the qualities they reject as (belonging to the) other.

This line of argument may be familiar as a typical poststructuralist manoeuvre, and part of my intention in writing this chapter is to argue that the poststructuralist influence on scholarship offers us a source of theoretical insight that remains largely untapped, at least in the UK, by nurses in their understanding of their own situation. I would like to stir up some interest among nurses in the specific tactics of discourse analysis, which I will describe later, as well as in poststructuralist thought as a whole. The analysis I will present here also draws upon poststructuralist literary theory, providing an alliance that underpins a powerful theoretical position from which to examine the discursive strategies used by nurses and managers not only in their argumentation but also in their self-understanding.

Nursing as a moral activity

The words of nurses that I will discuss in this chapter need to be understood in two contexts; the recent policy history of the UK National Health Service and the slightly more far-reaching history of nursing's professional genealogy. In Chapter 5, I offered an account of the NHS policy context along with some of the political and philosophical origins of these policies. In the present chapter, I will take two reflections on the impact of managerialism on nursing as a springboard to speak at a little more length about the 'problem' of nursing's 'moral' discourses.

Nursing, morality and self-sacrifice

Strong & Robinson, writing about the introduction of general management to the UK NHS in the mid-1980s, differentiated the new general managers' responses to nursing and medicine (Strong & Robinson 1990). A key difference that these authors identified in managers' approaches revolved around medicine's 'intimate links with science' that nursing appeared to lack. The managers quoted in their study caricatured nurses as submissive and ignorant, while their criticism of doctors centred around their 'excess of individualism'. Similarly, Walby & Greenwell (1994) present an analysis of both the difference and the conflict between nursing and medicine that is predominantly task-orientated, although, of course they acknowledge the immense institutional power base of medicine. They differentiate the impact of managerialism on the two occupations in terms of the relative autonomy of each, adopting a widely accepted, and stereo-typical, view of nursing as rigid, hierarchical and rule-bound.

Many who have championed nursing's modern development have looked to its early history for explanations of nursing's submissiveness and, if not ignorance, its lack of a conscious scientific basis for its activity. Nursing's history has involved a struggle between those who have promoted a discourse of nursing as a morally located activity and those who emphasised technical expertise and autonomy of practice, established professional characteristics. Although, of course, there is no reason why it could not be both, the search for the 'essential' meaning of nursing has tended to fall into this dualism. An emphasis on nursing's moral context involved considerable attention to the practi-tioner's own moral performance. Early nursing's failure to separate 'autonomy from altruism', according to Reverby, resulted in nurses accepting a duty to care but without contributing to how that care was constituted (Reverby 1987). Reverby also argues that Nightingale's understanding of nursing, and nurse training, as character develop-ment, a calling involving strict adherence to orders passed through a female hierarchy, led to an unempowering posture and to the reinforce-ment of the notion of separate spheres of activities for women and men:

> Duty remained the basis for nursing and … nurses found it difficult to achieve the collective transition out of a woman's culture of obligation into an activist assault on the structure and beliefs oppressing them.
>
> (Reverby 1987)

Such a collective attitude has been seen to 'legitimise men's right to supervise and superintend the behaviour of women' (Rafferty 1993, p. 51).

The intense scrutiny of nurses' moral performance in these early (and more recent) days seems to both reflect and reinforce an essen-tially moral understanding of nursing activity. For example, the prin-ciple of efficient surveillance, as it does in Bentham's Panopticon,* lies

---

*Jeremy Bentham (1748–1832), one of the founders of 'Utilitarianism', proposed an architectural design to solve the problem of efficient surveillance, for the prison or any other 'disciplinary' institution. It has become an emblem of a disciplinary age: 'at the periphery, an annular building; at the centre, a tower; this tower is pierced with wide windows that open onto the inner side of the ring; the peripheric building is divided into cells, each of which extends the whole width of the building; they have two windows, one on the inside, corresponding to the windows of the tower; the other, on the outside, allows the light to cross the cell from one end to the other. All that is needed, then, is to place a supervisor in a central tower and to shut up in each cell a madman, a patient, a condemned man, a worker or a schoolboy. By the effect of backlighting, one can observe from the tower, standing out against the light, the small captive shadows in the cells of the periphery … each actor is alone, perfectly individualised and constantly visible.' (Foucault 1977, p. 200).

at the heart of Nightingale's ward design. She argued that poor ward design contributed to lack of hospital discipline. In Nightingale's *Notes on Hospitals* (1883), discussed by Baly (1986), she records meticulous details of a ward layout which allows not only the penetration of the maximum of fresh air and light but also permits nurses to be under constant supervision. Even nurses' meals, she writes, ideally should be eaten in the ward scullery unless attended by the superintendent:

> The whole establishment must be so constructed that the probationers' dining rooms, day rooms, dormitories and the matron's residence and office must be put together and the probationers under the matron's immediate hourly direct inspection and control.

> (Nightingale 1865, cited in Baly 1988, p. 6)

Anne Marie Rafferty describes how in the last 40 years of the 19th century the emphasis in training objectives shifted from moral to professional. A new nursing elite looked to medicine for its inspiration in developing a model of professional organisation (Rafferty 1993). This involved the call for registration. Opponents of registration rejected claims for similarity and, by implication, intellectual and social parity with medicine. They argued that the medical emphasis was scientific and intellectual while 'by contrast, nursing was qualitatively different and "good" nursing could not be tested by examination' (Rafferty 1993, Rathbone 1892). Similar claims for an unquantifiability about nursing are sometimes raised today, though since the days of the 'internal market' and the NHS research and development strategy (DoH 1991), such a discourse has become less legitimate – and less commonly heard.

Nursing registration was discussed in a context where women's suffrage was high on the country's political agenda. 'The nurse question is the woman question,' said Mrs Bedford Fenwick (Rafferty 1993, p. 195). Nursing reformers saw their profession's struggle to be differentiated from and stand alongside the male bastion of medicine as part of women's wider struggle for equality. However, Rafferty argues that groups in nursing, keen to secure certain privileges adopted the same traditions advocated by those groups which they perceived as already having achieved success (Rafferty 1992, p. 33). The organisation of nursing history began to mirror that of medicine in its appeal to exemplary figureheads and foundational principles. Nutting & Dock, early historians of nursing, attempted to construct an illustrious history by appealing to the legitimacy of science to argue for the supreme status of 'caring' (Nutting & Dock 1907, p. 6). According to Russian zoologist Kropotkin, quoted by Nutting & Dock, Darwin was mistaken; it was in caring and cooperation, not combat and competition wherein lay the key to evolutionary success. Using this approach they attempted to form a (dubious) association between a universal characteristic and the professional activity of a particular group. This attempt to unite moral and scientific discourses (not to mention professional) is perilous. More contemporary versions of this kind of move include those by Leininger. Leininger writes:

> For more than three decades, it has been my theoretical posture that caring is the essence of nursing and the explanadum for health and well-being. It is also the explanadum for the survival of human cultures and civilisations.
>
> (Leininger 1990, p. 19)

Alistair MacIntyre (1985) argues that we live in the aftermath of the failure of the Enlightenment's project to justify and ground morality by appeals to reason (such as Kant's) and rationality (Utilitarianism he argues was one such failure).

NURSING AND MANAGERIALISM

Moving into more recent years, nursing's response to the reforms of the NHS during the 1980s and 1990s has been mixed. In the 1980s, the Royal College of Nursing mounted a high profile publicity campaign attacking the very notion of general management on the grounds that general managers lacked professional expertise and would perhaps be unduly financially orientated. It was clearly felt that general management would not be good for the interests of nursing. Later, such frontal attacks gave way to more pragmatic approaches, with the aim of retaining some influence over nurses in senior management. To the most recent wave of reforms, there was an initial apprehension. The RCN felt that the UK government's white paper *Working for Patients* (DoH 1989), in which the key principles of the reforms were set out, 'undermined the principles and effectiveness of the NHS and placed at risk most of the progress that had been made since 1948' (Butler 1992, p. 60). Speaking in 1992, former RCN General Secretary, Trevor Clay commented that he found it hard to welcome a market structure 'which deliberately forces a competitive ethos on nurses.'

He claimed that, by contrast, the values which underpin nursing are those of 'partnership, teamwork and collaboration' (Nursing Standard News 1992b). In the community health setting, where the fieldwork of this study is located, virtually every aspect of the reforms was seen as a possible threat to nursing numbers or its status or both (Lowe 1990, North & Porter 1991, Nursing Standard News 1992a, Prentice 1991). Many community nurses, particularly health visitors, whose role is based upon preventive activities, expressed concerns not only about how to 'package their care attractively for General Practitioners, self-governing Trusts, the NHS or even private organisations' but also how to quantify the 'unquantifiable' caring role of the nurse (Mason 1991). At other times nurses were urged to be pragmatic in their approach to the reforms (Nursing Times News 1990) while others argued that central aspects of the reforms were entirely in line with community nurses' desire to provide high-quality, locally responsive services. For one writer in the nursing press, adopting a so-called 'marketing philosophy' (not quite a 'market philosophy') was a question not so much of survival but more of promoting some of nursing's central values (Edwards 1994).

In summary, nursing's early history can be understood as a struggle between competing moral and scientifico-professional discourses. Recent NHS reorganisations, and the coming of the NHS research and development strategy, have challenged nursing's official bodies to re-enact this debate, coming down largely in favour of technical and professional accounts of nursing activity. What is interesting about the talk of nurses discussed in this chapter is its apparent rejection of these discourses in its emphasis on nursing as a moral activity.

INTRODUCTION TO THE ANALYTICAL APPROACH: A FOCUS ON TEXT

It is now time to give an account of the part that poststructuralism plays in this project.

Structuralism, semiotics and the 'turn to language'

The influence of structuralism and poststructuralism since their rise to prominence particularly in France in the 1960s and 1970s has led those from a range of disciplines including philosophy, sociology and psychology to place language at the forefront of their inquiry. Structuralism flourished in mid-century continental thought, but has roots in the work of Swiss linguist Ferdinand de Saussure (1857–1913), whose *Course in General Linguistics* was published posthumously in 1916 (first edition in English 1959, reprinted 1974).

De Saussure provided the insight that language can be thought of as a system of structural relations that precedes and is presupposed by any given utterance, that it can be looked at as a structure outside of time. He called his theory of language 'semiology'; the science of signs. De Saussure investigated the distinction between any particular concept such as 'dog', which he termed the *signified*, and the speech sound associated with it, the *signifier*. He called the combination of signified and signifier the *sign*. He suggested that the connection between any signifier and its signified was arbitrary. Not only are the speech sounds associated with certain concepts arbitrary – they vary from language to language – but, crucially, the concepts themselves are indeterminate. Using examples from different languages, De Saussure demonstrated that certain categories and distinctions are available to speakers of some languages but not to the speakers of others. 'The world can be conceptually partitioned in endless different ways' (Potter & Wetherell 1987, p. 25). It is a sign's place within a particular system, its difference from other signs, that gives it meaning. This is the idea that lies behind De Saussure's notion of a science of the signs used by societies. In this science, 'signs' would include not only language, but any realm to which meaning has been applied. Fashion, buildings and travel guides have been analysed in this spirit (Barthes 1972, 1985).

De Saussure emphasised, however, that while linguistic signs may be arbitrary, this does not mean that the individual has the ability to alter a sign once it has become established within a community. This shift from a concentration upon the individual, or 'decentring' of the individual, to the organising life of structures is a key move in structuralist thought.

Structuralism, with its 'timeless' or diachronic preoccupation, has been criticised for a lack of attention to history, culture, politics, the material world (Turner 1994) and how these forces may have influenced structures under study. Poststructuralism, and certainly the present study, attempts to avoid this limitation.

Structuralism, poststructuralism

Structuralist thought led, for a variety of reasons, some more perhaps to do with murky issues of academic politics than theory (Turner 1994), into what has been termed 'poststructuralism'. According to poststructuralism, language is a far less stable affair than the structuralists suggested, for example the search for the meanings of signs leads us not to definitive meanings but to other signs in an endless fashion. Secondly, meaning is dependent on context and open to endless citations in different contexts. (We may speak of 'art' or again of 'art and science', 'art' taking on a different meaning according to context.) Meanings, in a sense, are not and can never be, fully present within signs.

Some poststructuralists also argue that part of our western tradition has involved the search for the anchoring, unquestionable sign to which all our signs can be seen to point. Such a sign might be God, the World Spirit or the Self (Derrida 1982). This kind of sign needs to be 'beyond' and 'outside' of our system of signs as a 'first principle'. But first principles can always be deconstructed and shown to be products from *within* a particular system of meaning rather than what supports it or grounds it from the outside.

Poststructuralists argue that 'first principles' are commonly defined by what they exclude. In patriarchal societies, for example, man may be understood to be the founding principle and woman is the excluded opposite:

> Woman is the opposite, the 'other' of man: she is non-man, defective man, assigned a chiefly negative value in relation to the male first principle. But equally, man is what he is only by virtue of ceaselessly shutting out this other or opposite, defining himself in antithesis to it, and his whole identity is therefore caught up and put at risk in the very gesture by which he seeks to assert his unique, autonomous existence ... man therefore needs this other, even as he spurns it ... Not only is his own being parasitically dependent upon the woman and upon the act of excluding and subordinating her, but one reason why such exclusion is necessary is because she may not be quite so other after all. Perhaps she stands as a sign of something in man himself which he needs to repress, expel.
>
> (Eagleton 1983, p. 132, 133)

We might substitute 'rationality' and 'intuition' or even 'medicine' and 'nursing' for man and woman. The crucial link between poststructuralism and political struggle is that signs pass themselves off as 'natural', as the only credible or conceivable way of viewing the world. These signs are, by that token, authoritarian and ideological and can be shown to be just that – cultural constructions of particular groups, reflecting. Dale Spender (1980), looking at women, and Edward Said (1978, 1993), writing about people colonised by white western powers, have argued that such groups not only have their identity but the structure of existence defined for them by the language (as well as the brute power) of powerful outside groups. One area of enquiry that focuses on language and investigates how signs pass themselves off as 'natural' in particular situations or institutions is discourse analysis.

Discourse analyses

A great many approaches to text go under the name of discourse analysis (Potter & Wetherell 1987), from measurement-oriented analysis of the structures of a text (Renkema 1993), through analysis of conversation and turn-taking (Sacks et al 1974) to more broadly ideological studies (Thompson 1984). However, from a poststructuralist angle, I would argue that approaches to talk that concentrate on analysis of the structure of conversation with its turn-taking and other sequences or with producing 'models' of argumentation or numerical accounts of the reading process do not do justice to the inevitable ambiguity of texts. What I would like to emphasise and argue for is an analysis that investigates the link between knowledge, language and social and political power, an analysis that tries to make explicit the philosophical positions implicit in particular instances of talk. In this chapter I will use nurses' utterances as an example of the use of discourse to persuasive effect, as a representation of their interests.[†]

Parker suggests the following definition of discourse:

> Discourses do not simply describe the social world, they categorise it, they bring phenomena into sight. ... once an object has been elaborated in a discourse, it is difficult *not* to refer to it as if it were real. Discourses provide frameworks for debating the value of one way of talking about reality over other ways.
>
> (Parker 1992, pp. 4–5)

It is possible to move discourse analysis beyond linguistic concerns and see virtually the whole world as 'textual' in so far as it is understood

---

[†]For a fuller account of the theoretical origins of discourse analysis, see Potter & Wetherell (1987).

and given meaning by us: '[t]here is nothing outside of the text' (Derrida 1976, p. 158).

Foucault has argued that discourses are 'practices that systematically form the objects of which they speak' (Foucault 1972, p. 49). However, there is a particular kind of object – the subject – who either 'speaks, writes, hears or reads the texts discourses inhabit':

> A discourse makes available a space for particular types of self to step in. It addresses us in a particular way. When we discourse analyse a text, we need to ask in what ways, as Althusser (Althusser 1971) put it when he was talking about the appeal of ideology, the discourse is hailing us, shouting 'hey you there' and making us listen as a certain type of person.
>
> (Parker 1992, p. 9)

In the present research, for example, some managers spoke about the 'dead wood' in their trusts; a kind of talk that places us as taxpayers, or organisational members with a natural abhorrence of financial waste. On the other hand, discourses about 'patient/clients' inclines us to respond as compassionate, human individuals. Although the person or institution giving expression to a discourse may place themselves in a number of subject positions including the two above, this subject need not be a consistent one; it can change during the course of a text and can even appear to inhabit a number of spaces simultaneously.

THE ROYAL COLLEGE OF NURSING RESEARCH

As outlined in the introduction to the book and the previous chapter, the Royal College of Nursing undertook a longitudinal research study to examine the impact of the 1991 NHS reforms upon community health services. For the 'nursing' strand of the research, all the nurses employed in each participating area were asked to complete an anonymous questionnaire assessing job satisfaction. The main body of this questionnaire was numerical but nurses were also invited to add comments. These surveys started in April 1991 and were repeated once in each of the two subsequent years. The interviews with managers started in 1992 and were repeated in the two subsequent years. I also made detailed field notes during attendance at 48 meetings of nursing staff. The study design made a comparison of the views of the workforce and management possible.

Between one-third and one-half of responding nurses offered condensed statements of their values, often set in contrast to descriptions of rising forces that they saw within their organisations or in society as a whole. The strongly worded quotations included in this analysis are not atypical of these comments. Anger, frustration, outrage and bitterness were common. Comments that supported managerial perspectives and organisational change appeared, but were rare in the extreme.

The nurses' comments

The number of nurses who wrote comments during the 3 years of the study in the various organisations is given in Table 6.1. For the purposes of the analysis in this chapter, little distinction is drawn between different organisations and the years of the study. The comments varied in length; between one sentence and two sides of closely written text, attached to the original questionnaire.

Comments were made by nurses holding a wide variety of job titles in community settings; both those employed by individual GPs, including the then new fundholding GPs, and those employed within NHS trusts. Table 6.2 summarises the job titles of the nurses who commented. The 3 years of the study are combined. Middle managers were included in the study of job satisfaction as well as in the interview study of managers.

The questionnaire comments: how nurses talked about their work

Dualism; the nurse and the bureaucrat

This section deals with the dualistic way that nurses described themselves in relation to management and how they effected, by means of this rhetorical dualism, a claim for the moral supremacy of caring.

Table 6.1 Numbers of comments from trust areas

Trust	Year of survey			
	1	2	3	All
1	141	130	115	
2[a]	86			
3	54	57	44	
4	88	92	79	
Total	369	279	238	886

[a]Withdrew from study after year 1.

Table 6.2 Job titles of commenting nurses

Job title	Number
Practice nurse	198
Health visitor	177
District nurse	140
Trained hospital staff[a]	83
Nursing auxiliary	82
Enrolled nurse	60
Community staff nurse	41
Schools nurse	25
Middle managers	24
Others	56
Total	886

[a]One of the trusts managed a number of 'cottage' hospitals.

Criticism of administrators and managers is not a new thing in nursing (Mercer 1979). In the present study, nurses described how they saw management as having different priorities and values from themselves. They tended to express this with a series of 'us–them' dualisms. Many of the dualisms opposed 'care' to 'money' but other dualisms suggested different dimensions of the alienation many nurses described. The 'caring' side of the dualism was given a moral and epistemological privilege: not only was this discursive structure the means by which nurses adopted a position of moral superiority but the knowledge that it gave access to was described as of a more real and authoritative nature than the more abstracted knowledge associated with managers' reports and 'statistics'. This dense series of dualisms suggested how one aspect of nurses' subjectivity was constituted by a combining of discourses of moral value and of empiricism, an assertion of the privilege of the direct evidence of the senses. In some respects, their subjectivity was the mirror image of that adopted by managers who asserted the epistemology of the overview with its detachment that lent them an ability to penetrate to the reality of the situation. Managers also questioned the moral ability of some of their workforce to turn away from traditional methods of working and face 'realistic' financial constraints. In fact many nurses explicitly identified their work and values as 'traditional', while managers spoke of themselves as bringers of modernity and radical change. Such is the power of rhetoric that each group could present these opposing discourses in a way that we as reader might find equally appealing. Notable in many nurses' comments was the claim that the threat to 'caring values' was a *new* phenomenon and this too was reflected in the words of managers who took the recent NHS reforms as a central reference point in their worldview.

The rhetorical tone of a great many nurses' comments was of moral outrage. It could be that the format through which they were asked to respond encouraged a condensing of both the content and force of their views. However, a similar outrage often dominated the staff meetings that I attended where different constraints existed. Perhaps it is entirely consistent with the subject positions adopted by nurses and managers that managers should adopt the language of solidarity with their organisation, of control, of the rationality of the penetrating statement or observation and that field staff, lacking this organisational power and not using this vocabulary, had learnt to draw upon a moral discourse to characterise their subjectivity.

Caring, employment and exploitation

One key to understanding the texts of the nurses lies in the notion of split subjectivity. Nurses appeared to be constantly negotiating between a discourse of caring as morally worthwhile and intrinsically satisfying and an alternative discourse of exploitation in the workplace. The discursive tactic adopted to reconcile these two positions was that of the personal sacrifice, and, within this sacrifice, the exercise of individual judgement about standards of care could be understood as a point of resistance to the power of management to measure and control their activity.

First, we can look at how 'caring' was constructed in the texts from the 100 comments with relevance to this and then we can move on to consider ways in which constraints upon caring were understood and resisted.

Many nurses adopted the discourses of vocation and duty that more conspicuous voices in nursing have sought to downgrade in favour of more professionalised discourse (Kitson 1993). Nurses described caring in personal terms. They brought to this personal encounter a background in and personal commitment to helping and supporting and a belief that particular individuals had a need for as well as an entitlement to the service that they offered (a mixture of humanism and welfare discourses). Nurses appeared acutely aware that care could vary in quality and that good-quality caring demanded the vital ingredient of adequate time. Adequate resources and training were described as necessary by only a few. What constituted high-quality care was a matter of individual judgement, occasionally referred to as 'professional judgement', and the personal standards of the individual nurse. The outcome of good care was emotional satisfaction for both client/patient and for the nurse. However, descriptions where satisfaction was not the outcome tended to predominate. In these situations the outcome was stress and distress for the nurses involved. What prevented these high standards of care was generally lack of time. Nurses made a frequent distinction between their 'own time' and their paid working hours. The encroachment into their personal time of working activities was frequently cited as an example of the personal sacrifice that nurses offered in an attempt to avoid what they saw as poor-quality or incomplete care. Administrative duties, which were seen as the antithesis to care delivery, were frequently named as a cause of time constraints. The practicality of care delivery was contrasted with and seen to be under threat not only from management but from the profession's own leaders and educators with attempts to theorise or complicate it. Caring was constructed as an activity of high moral value and contrasted with financial concerns which were seen as less morally valuable if not morally suspect.

A personal commitment to care

Many nurses characterised their activities by appealing to a discourse of vocation which for a few nurses even crossed the boundary between the private and public realms. This had the effect of locating their orientation in primarily moral rather than occupational terms:

> I am doing the job I had always wanted to do, caring for people that needed caring or a helping hand …
>
> (Nursing auxiliary)

> Each day I aim to do my job to 100% of my capabilities to ensure my patients' well-being and happiness, and then return home to do the same for the rest of my family.
>
> (Practice nurse)

There were few references to professional training as a basis for practice. When it was referred to it tended to be used as an assertion of the legitimacy of direct care activity. In the quotation below, 'proper' and the slightly quaint 'etiquette' contrast with 'new fangled'. This move allows nursing training and practice to be associated with a tradition and propriety with which other, possibly administrative, activities can be contrasted as faddish and trivial. The purpose of nurse training is described in terms that persuade the reader of its direct and almost timeless quality and importance, 'care of the sick':

> ... I was trained for ... 'care of the sick' ... new fangled time wasters come between me and my proper nursing training and etiquette.

> (Marie Curie nurse)

The constitution of the needy

Caring centred around an encounter with people who, according to nurses' comments, also brought a personal attribute, or moral state, that of 'need'. Although nurses repeatedly conveyed the strongest sense of urgency regarding this need (see emphasis in the first quotation below), need also appeared, paradoxically, to be something that was detected and defined by nurses, as in the comments below and particularly in the argument that certain families 'need' 'professional support and guidance'. The discourse constructs the category of the needy patient:

> As a student I have more opportunity to spend longer time with patients/families, time that *they need*.

> (District nursing student – original emphasis)

> Approx. one-third of my caseload comprises of families of concern (various reasons) who need extra HV support and it is a constant struggle to provide them with the professional support/guidance which they need and are entitled to.

> (Health visitor)

Many writers referred to clients' and patients' 'right' or 'entitlement' to care, as in the second comment above. This had the effect of calling upon two distinct but linked discourses. One might be called a welfare discourse, with its echoes of the founding ethos behind the UK Welfare State. Within this discourse, entitlement has broad moral associations but can be considered a specific reference to formal entitlements linked to the payment of National Insurance contributions. The other might be termed a deontological discourse calling upon notions of the paramount importance of the human rights and value of each individual (Seedhouse 1993). Deontologists argue that each human life has an intrinsic value and that this value is not compromised or reduced by illness or disability. Because of this, essentially utilitarian arguments that are based upon setting measurable equivalents between the different benefits of health care, for example in the notion of QALYs (Maynard 1993) are rejected. Although no nurse made such arguments explicit in his or her comments, it could be argued that an implicit deontology characterised many comments and formed a contrast to the largely utilitarian thinking of the managers. It may be this fundamental difference in ethical stance that made nurses appear so irrational to managers whose overriding central task appeared to lie in determining equivalents and comparisons in the use of apparently fixed resources.

The vast majority of comments about caring described a situation of frustration rather than successful or satisfying care.

> [I am] always aiming to offer the patients in the care of my team a high standard of quality care. I am now struggling to continue my standard of care.
>
> (District nurse)

> Nurses desperately trying to maintain a high standard of care to patients ...
>
> (District nurse)

Judgement and resistance

Having made a convincing account of the moral basis and vocational commitment to deliver care, and having presented the forces militating against its delivery, nurses could then constitute decisions made about caring as originating from the realm of the personal and moral. It is this last move that so thwarted management in its drive for nurses to work from (so-called) rational, formalised decisions. It could be argued that this was the one point where nurses had the possibility to exercise power. The criteria for deciding quality and for decisions about care were nearly always described in the vocabulary of personal feeling and judgement:

> ... not able to give quality of care I think patient needs.
>
> (District nurse)

> I feel I don't have enough time to give patients the quality of nursing care which they deserve.
>
> (District nurse)

> I hope I give an extremely high standard of care.
>
> (Health visitor)

A contrasting note in strongly contrasting language was struck by the single nurse who spoke about formalised outcomes and linked standards of care with an organisational rather than personal initiative:

> Overall, trust status has centred thinking and improved standards of care with more emphasis on outcomes of care.
>
> (Health visitor)

Time: the personal sacrifice

Nurses often wrote about personal sacrifice of time worked to achieve what they considered to be adequate care. Nurses appeared to be almost forced to attempt a split subjectivity. As subjects within the discourse of caring as morally worthwhile, empowering and intrinsically satisfying, it would be inconsistent to complain about carrying work into hours beyond those which were financially rewarded; however, they also spoke of continued exploitation. Perhaps as a way of negotiating a position that accounted for both subjectivities, many adopted the discourse of sacrifice. This could act not only to intensify the moral value of their activities, because it gave evidence that their actions were not self-interested, but also to augment the injustice of their exploitation, because their moral sensitivity or agency rendered them particularly vulnerable to abuse. Within this subject position were a range of stances from frank anger:

> ... the worker can have given a lifetime of commitment ... and at the end of the day ... it is totally forgotten ...
>
> (Health visitor)

> Nurses are sick of being used and abused by the system.
>
> (Staff nurse)

to ambivalent stances apparent in these comments, which contained both acceptance and refusal to accept the situation:

> I give my patients 200% of quality work and my time. I would worry and feel unfulfilled if all the cost cutting is affecting their recovery and well-being. I hide my feelings.
>
> (District nurse)

> I spend a lot of my own personal time with pts. [patients] i.e. I always run late in order to give them the care they need – I don't mind – because I do have a lot of job satisfaction however – I should not *have* to regularly use my own time to give proper care.
>
> (Nursing auxiliary – original emphasis)

The personal terms in which nurses described decision-making lent little flexibility to the situation and little satisfaction as a point of resistance. Discussion during staff meetings that I attended reinforced the same sense:

One EN (Enrolled nurse) said she visited a woman today who had lost both her husband and daughter within six weeks. 'All I had time to do was to dress her leg ulcer. I could have spent all morning with her.' 'All there is time for', said the manager, 'is the nitty-gritty stuff. All the frills that we were trained to do, don't get done.'

(Field notes November 1992, Trust 4)

It is possible that the locality manager who speaks uses the term 'the frills' to describe what most nurses would consider the essential aspects of their work out of a jaded acceptance that these have already been effectively marginalised.[‡]

The moral value of caring contrasted with financial concerns

A number of nurses drew strong contrasts between the moral value of caring for people and the lesser or even dubious consideration for financial matters with which they associated senior managers. The first year's comments regarding this were more frequent and vehement in their language than those of subsequent years.

This dualism allowed commenters, who identified their concerns with caring and who had also detailed the personal sacrifices entailed in delivering care, to take the moral 'high ground'. In this way they identified their interests with those of their patients:

The world of business has definitely taken over, and as well as not giving as much time to the patents as we would like, there is a lack of caring for us as the carers.

(District nurse)

Numbers, finances and balancing books is becoming more important than people. The organisation doesn't really *care* for its workforce.

(Health visitor – original emphasis)

One nurse expressed an uncompromising view that can be seen to underlie many of the comments made in the first year. This comment, in which the need of the human individual is described as completely overriding any financial concern, can be understood as a distillation of the deontological view mentioned previously:

I think we should look at the care services available first rather than discussing how much money it will incur. Working within budget policy is unapplicable and inappropriate in caring for elderly/mentally handicapped and or physically handicapped clients.

(Staff nurse)

[‡]The unique and often painful predicament of the 'middle' manager merits further discussion.

Nursing subjecthood and the operation of power

This chapter has brought poststructuralist notions of discourse and subjectivity to bear upon the words of nurses working in the first 3 years of the reformed UK NHS (that is, the 1991 reforms). It has attempted to take forward an understanding of the difficulty experienced by nursing clinicians within a National Health Service that is increasingly characterised by the rationality of managerial control. Poststructuralist accounts of the operation of power have made an analysis possible that moves beyond understanding power as simple oppression by one group of another. Deborah Lupton, for example, poses certain key questions in her exploration of the character of 'critical discourse analysis':

> how do individuals take up, negotiate, or resist discourse and how is resistance generated and sustained? What are the constraints to taking up subject positions? How are the individuals interpellated, or 'hailed' by discourses – how do they recognise themselves within?
>
> (Lupton 1995)

It has been possible to argue that many nurses in this study negotiated a subjectivity that was forged out of conflicting discourses of caring and exploitation within their employing organisations. In this sense, the application of managerial power gave rise to this particular subjectivity. However, within this apparently highly constrained situation, nurses attempted to hold on to a sense of autonomy by linking their professional judgement with their sense of moral agency. The result of this was a position characterised by self-sacrifice. The exercise of individual judgement at the site of caring was understood as a point of resistance to managerial power or at least a possible point of such resistance as in many such instances nurses described being frustrated in their exercise of judgement by the constraints of time. Nurses created a subjectivity for themselves that contrasted with the avowed rationality of their managers.

Since I first began to speak about these ideas in public, it has been pointed out to me that the identification of nurses in direct care roles with moral agency and of managers with 'rationality' tends to imply a homogeneity and a stability within the two groups. Such an analysis also does not acknowledge those occasions when nurses drew upon utilitarian notions, often by arguing that money spent on 'another glossy brochure from the Department of Health' could have funded a particular number of extra nursing posts. There is also the danger that characterising the strongly utilitarian strands in the discourse adopted by managers as a form of rationality fails to take account of utilitarianism as an approach, albeit misguided (MacIntyre 1985), to answering essentially moral problems, such as how to use (supposedly fixed and hence) scarce resources. While the account of nurses' comments I have offered here provides a useful insight into the effect of powerful discourses, it is important to remember that we should be loath to fix nurses, managers, or any other group, into rigid positions.

REFERENCES

Althusser L 1971 For Marx. Allen Lane, London
Baly M 1986 The Nightingale reform and hospital architecture. History of Nursing Group at the Royal College of Nursing Bulletin 11: 1–7
Baly, M 1988 Florence Nightingale and the nursing legacy. Croom Helm, London
Barthes R 1972 Mythologies. Granada, Frogmore
Barthes R 1985 The fashion system. Cape, London
Butler J 1992 Patients, policies and politics: before and after 'Working for patients'. Open University Press, Milton Keynes
De Saussure F 1974 Course in general linguistics. Fontana, London
Department of Health (DoH) 1989 Working for patients. Cmd. 555 HMSO, London
Department of Health (DoH) 1991 Research for health; a research and development strategy for the NHS. HMSO, London
Derrida J 1976 Of grammatology. Johns Hopkins University Press, Baltimore
Derrida J 1982 White mythology: metaphor in the text of philosophy. In: Margins of philosophy. Wheatsheaf Harvester, Hemel Hempstead, pp 207–272
Eagleton T 1983 Literary theory: an introduction. Blackwell, Oxford
Edwards J 1994 How to sell your services in the NHS. Primary Health 4(1): 6–8
Foucault M 1972 The archaeology of knowledge. Routledge, London
Foucault M 1977 Discipline and punish. Penguin, Harmondsworth
Kitson A (ed) 1993 Nursing: art and science. Chapman and Hall, London
Leininger M 1990 Historic and epistemologic dimensions of care and caring with future directions. In: Stevenson J S, Tripp-Reimer T (eds) Knowledge about care and caring. American Academy of Nursing, Kansas City, MO, pp. 19–31
Lowe R 1990 Defending your territory. Nursing Standard 4(43): 50
Lupton D 1995 D & S forum: postmodernism and critical discourse analysis. Discourse and Society 6(2): 301–304
MacIntyre A 1985 After virtue. A study in moral theory. Duckworth, London
Mason C 1991 Project 2000: a critical review. Nursing Practice 4(3): 3
Maynard A 1993 The economics of rationing health care. In: Tunbridge M (ed) Rationing of health care in medicine. Royal College of Physicians, London, ch 1
Mercer G 1979 The employment of nurses. Nursing labour turnover in the NHS. Croom Helm, London
Nightingale F 1865 Letter to H. Bonham Carter. Greater London Records Office HI/ST/NC 18(6)
Nightingale F 1883 Notes on hospitals. Longman Green, London
North N, Porter E 1991 All change ahead. Nursing Times 87(3): 57–59
Nursing Standard News 1992a Move to defuse practice nurses' fears over GPs. Nursing Standard 6(19): 6
Nursing Standard News 1992b News. Nursing Standard 6(49): 13
Nursing Times News 1990 Hancock urges positive outlook on reforms; speech at Primary Health Care Conference, November 1990. Nursing Times 86(45): 6

Nutting M, Dock L 1907 A history of nursing: the evolution of nursing systems from the earliest times to the foundation of the first English and American training schools. G P Putnam's, London

Parker I 1992 Discourse dynamics: critical analysis for social and individual psychology. Routledge, London

Potter J, Wetherell M 1987 Discourse and social psychology; beyond attitudes and behaviour. Sage publications, London

Prentice S 1991 What will we find at the market? Health Visitor 65(1): 9–11

Rafferty A M 1992 Historical perspectives. In: Robinson K, Vaughan B (eds) Knowledge for nursing practice. Butterworth-Heinemann, Oxford

Rafferty A M 1993 Decorous didactics: early explorations in the art and science of caring c. 1860–90. In: Kitson A (ed) Nursing: art and science. Chapman and Hall, London, pp 48–84

Rathbone W 1892 Evidence to the select committee of the House of Lords on metropolitan hospitals. Parliamentary Papers XIII.I(xci). HMSO, London

Renkema J 1993 Discourse studies: an introductory textbook. John Benjamins, Amsterdam

Reverby S 1987 A caring dilemma: womanhood and nursing in historical perspective. Nursing Research 36(1): 5–11

Sacks, H, Schegloff E, Jefferson G 1974 The simplest systematics for the organisation of turn-taking in conversation. Language 50: 697–735

Said E 1978 Orientalism. Pantheon, New York

Said E 1993 Culture and imperialism. The world, the text and the critic. Chatto and Windus, London

Seedhouse D 1993 Ethics: the heart of health care. John Wiley, Chichester

Spender D 1980 Man made language. Routledge and Kegan Paul, London

Strong P, Robinson J 1990 The NHS under new management. Open University Press, Milton Keynes

Thompson J 1984 Studies in the theory of ideology. Polity Press, Cambridge

Turner T 1994 Bodies and anti-bodies: flesh and fetish in contemporary social theory. In: Csordas T (ed) Embodiment and experience. The existential ground of culture and self. Cambridge University Press, Cambridge, pp 27–47

Walby S, Greenwell J 1994 Medicine and nursing. Professions in a changing health service. Sage, London

Interests and their realignment: managing medicine

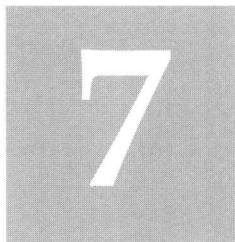

Joanna Latimer

7

■ **CONTENTS**

Introduction   163
Interests   164
  Incurring change through
   the translation of
   interests   165
Health care systems under
  strain   166
Throughput: a new strategic
  value   168

Patients: a target to be
  managed   170
The bedside as a site of
  exclusion   172
The pea lady   174
Discussion   179
Conclusion   180
References   182

INTRODUCTION

> It's all about throughput these days
>
> (Staff Nurse, cited in Latimer 1996)

> Apparently what's wrong with the NHS is older people. If the over 60s would just disappear, the rest of us would never have to wait for a bed again ....
>
> (Philips 1997)

This chapter and the following one address the question of how it is that participants in health care systems fall into line with a prevailing set of interests. The specific example with which the chapters are concerned is how increasing inpatient throughput has become a dominant concern for health care practitioners in acute health care environments during the 1980s and early 1990s. It is argued that throughput has become the dominant strategic value through which to manage medicine and health care systems because it has, through both formal and informal accountability relations (Munro 1996), become integrated with the performance of positive identities in health care environments. At the same time, increasing throughput has meant that some practitioners may have had to realign their understandings of what patients need and shift the focus and extent of their own responsibilities.

The current chapter opens with a discussion of the nature of interests. The ways in which the interests of doctors in British health care contexts have been aligned with managerial objectives concerned with increasing patient throughput is then elaborated. A particular effect is to focus doctors on the time (and therefore the resources) patients may take up, and on the assessment of patients in terms of their susceptibility to treatment and care, and therefore to helping doctors accomplish positive medical and managerial outcomes. It is suggested that managerial objectives over increased patient throughput may have had unintended consequences, such as the enhancement of the bedside as a 'site of exclusion'. The chapter concludes that rather than thinking of managerial and medical objectives as competing with older, 'more ethical' concerns of the medical professions over cure and care of individuals, or over public good, there has been a complicity between managerial and (some) medical objectives over the importance of particular forms of knowing and action.

INTERESTS

Interests are usually thought of as what 'lie behind' (Marcus & Fischer 1986), of what, perhaps, secretly and covertly motivate actors. Interests can also be considered as fixed, or as something chosen, connected to drawing power, or some other valued property, to self or group. Interests can also be considered as socially constructed: like values, they are something we cannot help *having*, because they go with our class, gender or some other social identity. Within the sociology of opposition, interests are political, associated with groups, such as 'the medical profession' or 'health visitors', as aggregates of individuals with common political concerns. In these circumstances, interests are promoted on behalf of the group, or of the good of others, like 'patients' or 'local communities'. These groups may take on the status of movements, and may attempt to persuade or even coerce others to act in ways which will achieve the movements' interests. To have an interest is, thus, to be biased, partial and, perhaps, calculating.

I do not want to refute these notions of interest, I want to hold on to their cumulative resonance. But I do want to preserve an idea of interests as *concerns*. In this way, I am suggesting that interests do not necessarily just lie in the domains of the calculative and the political as separate from the ethical, as some kind of sacrosanct space. Rather, I want to stress how interests are also connected to the ethical lives of social actors. Within this view, the conduct of social actors is not separate from, but is enwrapped with their interests.

Incurring change through the translation of interests

Latour (1991) gives a simple example of how it is possible for a Parisian hotelier to change the practices of his guests, or some of them at least. The concern of the hotelier is to stop his clients from leaving the hotel with their room keys: he wants the keys to remain on hotel premises. First, the hotelier instructs the receptionists to tell the guests on their arrival that they must leave the key at reception when they go out. A few more guests begin to do this. He then puts up a notice inscribed with a reminder to guests to leave their keys at reception. A slightly greater percentage of guests leave their keys at reception on leaving the hotel. Then the hotelier has large weights made and attaches these to the keys: many more guests leave their keys at reception, because now, rather than carry around a heavy weight with them all day in Paris, it is in their interests to leave the key at reception. Thus, the hotelier accomplishes a translation of the interests of his clients. Through complex processes of alignment he enrols them in his project: he aligns the verbal request, with the notice inscribed with an injunction, with the materiality of the weight attached to the end of the key. By this time, for guests who presumably want to travel around Paris sight-seeing, shopping, meeting a lover, or just on business, the key becomes something which intrudes on their concerns, as say a concern to minimise the strain and promote easy mobility.

This story helps us to see how interests or concerns are both mixed and mutable. Interests can be translated to incur a shift in the ways in which social actors order or prioritise their concerns: at the beginning of the story the guests were perhaps in a rush to get on and enjoy their visit, so that it was in their interests to forget the key, not to waste time queuing to hand it in at reception, while by the end of the story they remember the key and take that little time to deposit it because it is cumbersome, and may infringe on their objectives, a pleasurable stay in Paris. There are, then, particular *pre*configurations which make the realignment of the guests' interests possible (the enjoyment of their stay in Paris, for example), in favour of the hotelier. Because his move is to play on just that, their interest in being in Paris, he can accomplish a power effect, where this is understood not as domination or coercion, but where an individual or group 'attempt to impose themselves and their definition of the situation on others' (Callon 1986, p. 196).

The hotelier produces a change in the behaviour of other social actors, which is in his interests, but to do this he makes the change also in their interests by playing on something which is *already present*. He does not therefore simply change their interests, but incurs a realignment: the weight incurs a translation* of their interests in favour of his own. So there is not simply a *diffusion* of interests for change to occur; for changes in conduct to be effective there has to be a translation of interest. Whatever change is afoot needs to appear as in the interests of social actors, so that social actors take up any new strategy, device or programme, enrol it and in turn be enrolled by it to form a network of interests. But, and this is a critical aspect, the translations which occur are the effects of the particular configurations with which the social actor(s) is associated: the meanings interpreted for artefacts, the identities being constituted, the organising being accomplished and the other matters of interest involved.[†]

HEALTH CARE SYSTEMS UNDER STRAIN

The British health services at the end of the 1970s and beginning of the 1980s began to no longer appear as the most innovative (Loveridge & Starkey 1992) and remarkable health care system in the world, the pride of Britain, but as a system under 'strain' (Giddens 1984). Some commentators stress how pressure arose from a new kind of 'examination' of the health service: this new kind of examination came from the government's use of accounting technologies

---

*Latour (1986, p. 267) gives the following account of translation: 'the spread in time and space of anything – claims, orders, artefacts, goods – is in the hands of people; each of these people may act in many different ways, letting the token drop or modifying it, or deflecting it, to betraying it, or adding to it, or appropriating it.'

† The other point which Latour is stressing is the human–non-human relation: sometimes it is the non-human, such as the weight at the end of the key, which is (presumed) to be capable of incurring such a translation of interests and consequent changes in behaviour.

to examine the health services from a managerial perspective (Broadbent et al 1991). The main criticism was that the health services were inefficient, and that costs had to be contained. It was argued that costs could be contained by making existing services more efficient because then they would become more effective. One of the supporting claims was that *patients* were dissatisfied with the service: they had to wait too long for consultation, investigations and treatment, as well as put up with services more geared to the interests of a self-serving medical profession, or to the routinised practices of an overblown bureaucracy and an unresponsive nursing workforce.

The great challenge was how to detribalise and modernise the health services (Hunter 1994). The key to this was to make doctors more accountable, not to each other, but to managers and accountants (Broadbent et al 1991), not in terms of clinical outcomes, but in terms of cost and time. Quality of clinical practice has been held separate from service outcomes, and while there was increased pressure upon practitioners from the medical, nursing and social work disciplines to justify their practices (Walton 1986), clinical practice has until very recently remained a responsibility internal to each profession or between the professions (Latimer 1996). In contrast, efficiency has been made integral to the performance of doctors, both in terms of individual consultant contracts, and the introduction of contractual performance indicators such as completed consultant episodes, and, in terms of the performance of trusts and contractual performance targets, such as length of waiting times and cost of services. Thus a 'business ethos' has partly been instituted through introducing contractual forms of accountability (Laughlin 1996). Instituting contractual forms of accountability rather than 'communal' forms of accountability based on relations of trust (Laughlin 1996), can also be considered as an effect of a wider movement which undermines notions of the 'public good' (Clarke 1996). Further, activities undertaken in the name of social goods can be effaced because they are almost impossible to justify in terms of accounting technologies (Cooper 1988).

It is very difficult to say what or who was behind the refiguring of the health services as somehow cumbersome, over-bureaucratised, inequitable[‡] and in need of 'rationalisation' (see also Dingwall et al

---

[‡] I have in mind the attack on the London teaching hospitals: refigured no longer as centres of excellence from which knowledge, skill and acculturation could radiate out to the provinces, but as privileged and elitist centres of medical power.

1988, Strong & Robinson 1990). For some commentators there was demand coming from the 'public' (e.g. Walton 1986) for public services and industries to be made more accountable, while for other commentators, the Government was merely enrolling the notion of the public in their war against the professions, and against medicine in particular.

THROUGHPUT: A NEW STRATEGIC VALUE

The reformation of the health services can be understood, then, as putting into play two important strategies. First, rather than attempting to remove or erode doctors' overall responsibility for patient care, by enrolling doctors in managerial objectives through linking their performance to service rather than clinical outcomes, these strategies have attempted to preserve doctors' overall accountability for patient treatment and care, at the same time as they erode doctors' discretion.

Increased emphasis on accountability, and the individuation of accountability for service outcome measures, focuses scrutiny on each employee as an individual. Drawing on Foucault (1978), Rose & Miller (1992) argue that such accountability strategies enable a 'governmentality effect'. A governmentality effect is accomplished by those strategies and technologies which exercise the *self*-discipline of the individual in the attainment of objectives calculated elsewhere. Rose & Miller suggest the governmentality effect as a way of conceiving power as not 'so much a matter of imposing constraints' as of 'making up citizens capable of bearing a kind of regulated freedom' (p. 174). Individuals are not merely seen as the 'subjects of power', but as playing 'a part in its operations' (Rose & Miller 1992, p. 174). To facilitate this governmentality effect, calculation is centralised at the same time as it appears to grant more autonomy.

Second, and critically, by making service outcomes dependent upon the notion of patient throughput, doctors as the prime movers within health care contexts, can be focused on the *speed* with which patients can be got through the system. In this way managerial strategies have been directed at exploiting what already pre-existed: namely, the dominance of medical authority.

Critically, however, this strategy has been legitimated with claims that it is in the interests of the 'greatest number', not as a collective, but as aggregates of individuals as consumers. The Patient's Charter

(DoH 1991) signifies this legitimation: (in theory) reducing the time someone has to be 'in' the apparatus increases throughput, and thereby enables more consumers to access facilities and resources. This equation relies of course upon the preconception that practice was inefficient, that time was somehow being wasted on unnecessary procedures or activities, and that it will be practitioners themselves who will overcome these as obstacles to efficiency and service effectiveness. So speeding up throughput is represented as in the interests of patients reconstituted as the consumers of health care, who want *more* timely access and availability.

To cross-check whether services live up to consumer or user expectations, patient satisfaction surveys and patients' complaints are also used as service outcome measures, and accompany throughput targets as instruments through which to assess service efficiency and effectiveness. Critically, as Clarke (1996) notes, underpinning arguments for practices with claims that they are in the public interest or the interests of individual patients, the recourse of doctors and nurses in the past, have been made 'venal'. In their place:

> the legitimate forms of representing the public are now dominated by the 'mandate' of the national government at the centre and the technologies of customer surveys at the periphery. In place of the presumptions of 'trust' associated with old public service ethics, the relationships of public service have been increasingly formalised through contractual mechanisms, monitoring,§ and both financial and 'performance' audits.
>
> (Clarke 1996, p. 78)

Increasing throughput can therefore be taken to be a 'strategic value' (Munro 1992), through which to harness doctors to organisational goals and drive change. Because contractual accountability incorporates notions of complete consultant episodes, it has (theoretically) been made in doctors' interests to seek for, encourage, and permit practices and procedures which help to process patients more

---

§ Bloomfield et al (1992) have studied how responsibility accounting systems (resource management) work in relation to monitoring medical practice from a financial perspective. These kinds of systems, they suggest: 'construct and make visible significant aspects of organisational reality ... making possible new or more penetrating forms of organisational practice – such as Medical Audit. At the same time, a responsibility accounting system develops standards of behaviour such that "normal" practice cannot only be defined, but also measured, and deviations noted. What is also implied is that what is rendered visible, measured, and rewarded, gains legitimacy. Conversely, that which is not recognised by the formal system is often neither rewarded nor legitimate.' (p. 199).

quickly, or indeed find ways to exclude those patients who may be hard to get through the apparatus quickly *and* successfully. Thus, contractual accountability (should) help to enrol doctors in the managerial agenda of increased efficiency through reducing inpatient lengths of stay and increasing throughput.

However, I want to suggest that this particular re-formation of the health services has been attempted because it already resonated with the interests of the medical profession, not as aggregates of individuals with political interests, but with the medical profession as a discipline, which itself relies on the accomplishment of a particular kind of disciplined space.

PATIENTS: A TARGET TO BE MANAGED

The managerial reforms which have put into play a new strategic value, increased patient throughput, are aimed at the elimination of work which cannot be shown to have clear objectives and which does not lead to measurable outcomes. This brings with it the issue of reducing 'turnaround' times. Through contractual accountability, the Patient's Charter, and other devices, doctors' activities can be harnessed to organisational goals. Critically, however, these arrangements refigure the patient–professional relation because they rely on making *patients* the target to be managed, not by managers, but by practitioners as the managers of care: patients re-emerge as needing to be 'processed'.

I want to suggest that patients had already begun to be grouped in relation to their 'process-ability', prior to introduction of more explicit performance indicators, and the pseudo-marketisation of the health services. In what follows I draw on discourses concerned with the health care of ill older people because these help to illustrate how the need for managing patient care, or processing patients, had emerged as one response to the problem of increasing patient throughput *prior* to the introduction of management technologies such as contractual accountability. Indeed, it appears that the main drivers of such a focus were doctors in acute and geriatric medicine (e.g. Bouchier & Williamson 1982).

As already stated in Chapter 1, trends in health care organisation in Britain during the mid-1970s through to the 1980s were being driven by the need to 'rationalise' health service resources (Dingwall et al

1988). One feature of this was to focus on rate of bed occupancy, and lengths of stay for patients. The elderly were supposed to account for about half the population of patients within the acute sector (DHSS 1981) and, critically, older people were identified as taking longer to get out of hospital than younger adults, particularly older women and patients aged 75 and over (DHSS 1981, Scottish Hospital Inpatient Statistics). This gave rise to the notion of 'bed blocking' and of older people as potential 'bed-blockers' (Barker et al 1985, Coid & Crome 1986, Donaldson 1983, McArdle et al 1975, Rubin & Davies 1975, Seymour & Pringle 1982).

In this way older people were grouped together. They could be assembled into a group through the ways in which they were made visible as having particular characteristics. However, the discourse concerning older people and their care in the acute sector of the health services does not simply portray different views of reality but constitutes a discourse which reveals and articulates 'dimensions utilised to produce classifications and thus produce groups and relations' (Deetz 1992, p. 29). Rather than having medical problems, which could be resolved through the expertise of acute physicians, older people were figured as having more complex troubles, which were less susceptible to straightforward medical treatment and diagnosis. These complex troubles included multiple and chronic health problems, and health needs which had associated functional and psychosocial aspects. Longer lengths of stay in hospital were therefore attributed to the complexity of older people's troubles, and contingent poor assessment and care management, rather than simply to inappropriateness.

Thus, although statistically the older a person is the more likely he or she is to become ill, older people became a distinct category of patient, or potential patient, which was linked negatively with time, given the pressure to rationalise the health services by making them more efficient. An older person, therefore, could be seen to pose a possible *impediment* to the effective and efficient management of the acute sector, and to the increasing pressure on doctors to make visible the effectiveness of their practices (see also Walton 1986). It is much more difficult to accomplish medical objectives of diagnosis, treatment and cure in the complex environment of the older body. So, statistically, older people constituted as potential bed-blockers become a risk, not to themselves, but to doctors, because they may induce failures over throughput and over the continuous accomplishment of a pure, heroic and unadulterated medicine, unpolluted by the social; individually, ill or disabled older people are refigured, not as the objects of care or cure, but as targets, to be managed.

THE BEDSIDE AS A SITE OF EXCLUSION

Alternative and innovative arrangements were sought by many involved in the health care of elderly people. Among these alternatives were the use of community hospitals (North & Hall, unpublished work, 1984), special admissions and assessment wards for older people (Donaldson 1983), geriatrician input into general wards (Bouchier & Williamson 1982, Burley et al 1979, Grimley-Evans 1983) and augmented home care (Currie et al 1979). Innovations included implementation of special assessment tools, educational programmes and systems for nursing in an acute medical environment (see for example, Hulter Asberg 1986) and in special geriatric assessment wards (see for example, Bachman et al 1987).

In retrospect it can now be argued that what was set in motion was a massive reorganisation of health services to take account of the 'problem' of increasing numbers of ill or disabled older people, who had been identified as having the potential to block the flow through the beds. These discussions not only raise issues of responsibility and care with respect to acutely ill older people, but also contribute to how older people can be seen within the health services as potential 'bed-blockers' and how new experts, with their associated discourses and practices are required to alleviate/prevent this situation.

I now want to discuss how practitioners in one specific setting, an acute medical unit in a large and prestigious British teaching hospital in 1986–1987, both enrolled, and were enrolled in, managerial concerns over increasing throughput in the ways in which they conducted the care of people aged 75 and over. The study is discussed more fully in the Introduction, pp. 19–20.

At ward level, reducing length of stay and increasing throughput as an organisational strategy was never made explicit, nor was it formally connected to any one individual's performance. Rather, there was continuous pressure exerted on nurses and doctors alike through the ways in which the hospital was organised and through the activities of people, such as nursing officers, medical registrars and bed coordinators, who had come to be responsible for monitoring the bedstate (the numbers of empty and occupied beds). Each unit was responsible for taking emergency admissions from the accident and emergency department on its 'waiting day', but a problem with bed management had emerged over time, so that there was continuous pressure on staff over the matter of the availability of empty beds. At the beginning of the field study ward staff were presented with the demand for empty beds more frequently. As one Sister put it to me:

... we (the sisters) have all been given the message from the Community Medicine Specialist that when every fourth waiting day comes we are to have 10 beds empty.

Previously, it emerged, each unit had 'waited' every seventh day, and therefore had to have beds available every seventh day. This was then reduced to every sixth day and then, just prior to the current study, every fourth day. This gradual reduction in the time between being on take or waiting, meant that staff had to get patients through their wards faster. This increase in the pressure for the disposal of patients seemed to have several contingencies. First, nurses and doctors and others were more and more focused on *patient assessment*, not just in relation to present need, but in relation to future discharge: all patients were, from the moment they came into the hospital, observed, and judged continuously in relation to their capability, and their mobility, for their potential for movement, through the beds and out. Second, in order (perhaps) to accomplish greater efficiency in relation to patient assessment, and in acknowledgement (perhaps) of the complexity of some older patients' problems which might mean that some need would persist beyond discharge, the hospital had introduced geriatric consultation, and a system of multidisciplinary patient conference for all those people admitted to the acute wards over the age of 65. Third, an overnight admission and medical assessment unit had been opened, so that some patients could be thoroughly observed and assessed, prior to full admission to the hospital. This gave the opportunity for some patients to be transferred to more 'appropriate settings' than an acute unit, for example to a geriatric unit, or even to return home under the care of the GP with community support. Fourth, under circumstances where a patient was figured as a potential blockage to the flow through the beds, staff deployed practices which enabled a shift in the ways in which the older person's troubles could be accounted for, so that his or her needs were refigured as inappropriate to an acute medical domain (Latimer 1997). These practices drew on the personal, social and functional histories of older patients, made much more readily available through the proactive assessment practices of nurses, doctors and geriatricians. Indeed, elsewhere I have argued that with nursing and geriatric assessment, the biographical, social, economic and emotional lives of patients could be surveyed, to make available material with which to contextualise their troubles as not medical, but as chronic and due to the effects of biological decline, or as due to their social situation (Latimer 1998).

Thus, reducing length of stay and thereby increasing throughput was, partly, accomplished by practitioners modifying both what counts as a need and what is thought to be appropriate care and treatment within an acute medical unit: at the same time as they had extended their practices, to include geriatric assessment and surveillance of patients' psychosocial and functional lives, they also constituted classes of patient (Latimer 1997) which meant that some patients could now be excluded as inappropriate to the acute medical domain. In this way the bedside had become not just the space from which to administer and observe the sick body, but a 'site of exclusion'. To illustrate this point, I now turn to a ward round, during which a patient who has been in the hospital for 3 days, is turned round from being an appropriate patient for admission to an acute medical ward, to someone who can be discharged home.

The pea lady

To help exemplify these points, extracts from a ward round concerned with Mrs Marsh, are now analysed. It is 3 days after Mrs Marsh's admission to hospital; she is wearing a hospital gown and dressing-gown, and is sitting up in a chair by her bed in Bay 2.

The Ward Round comes into Bay 2. All the doctors are dressed in white coats. There are nine people involved plus myself, also in a white coat, and the Ward Sister in a white uniform dress with a white hat. The other important actor is the notes trolley, wheeled in by the resident.

Imagine 11, white-coated figures, coming to rest around one central figure, the consultant, also dressed in a white coat, possibly at the notes trolley or around that other artefact, the patient. This is a spectacle, which helps magnify *medical knowledge*; the knowledge that is inscribed in the notes, inscribed in the doctors, busy 'writing' (Latimer 1994) the patient, inscribed in the Sister who stands behind the others, taking her notes and rearranging curtains and bedclothes.

Sister, the doctors and the medical students are standing around the notes trolley and the consultant physician, who cuts the central figure.

Resident: (to Consultant) Mrs Marsh (indicates patient) – the pea lady.

Consultant: Is she new?

Resident: She came in the day before yesterday. (He reads from the notes and looks up at the Consultant as he speaks – he speaks quietly – confidentially – the others stand around.) Essentially she swallowed a pea at lunch time and became increasingly wheezy by the evening. By 8 o'clock she was very breathless and so 'phones her GP who sent her in here. She settled with nebulisers [a bronchodilation treatment for patients with bronchospasm and asthma]. She's been having daily physio'. Her drug history – she's on warfarin [an anticoagulant] – she's had a number of DVTs [deep vein thromboses or blood clots] in the past – but no pulmonary emboli [blood clots in the arteries leading to the lungs] (the Consultant is listening intently). She's on tamoxifen [a mild form of oral chemotherapy given for the treatment of breast cancer] for a lump in her breast but I can't find it.

Consultant: Have you got the old notes to see what goes on there?

Resident: No.

Consultant: (looks at the Registrar) Let's get hold of the old notes and check up on what's happening here (turns back to Resident).

Resident: There's some old myocardial ischaemia [damage to the heart muscle suggesting prolonged angina or an old heart attack], with some failure – she's fine – she lives alone. On systems inquiry she has some ankle swelling. She is apyrexial [without fever] and she has a ….

Consultant: (interrupts) So there is nothing of serious note on inquiry?

Resident: No.

At a distance, this seems to be a 'properly conducted' medical exchange: the resident presents the evidence in a quiet and confidential manner and the consultant checks that all that should be done is being done. As a managerial device the ward round constitutes a form of inspection and audit, of both doctors' work and aspects of nurses' work.

But on looking again there is more going on. The resident calls Mrs Marsh the 'pea lady', a strange metaphoric device. Doctors and nurses frequently call patients by their medical parts ('the appendectomy', 'the MI', 'the bunion') but Mrs Marsh is not referred to in this way, which would at least figure her as 'medical'. Rather, she is being figured through metaphorical reference to another, quite different domain: a pea, vegetable matter. And, further, the resident says she *swallowed* a pea and then became breathless, hours later, thus requiring a doctor. An ambiguity is brought into play here. Swallowing is the *normal* thing that should be done with a pea, no breathlessness should result. He then says that since she came to hospital she has had very limited treatment. The X-rays and ECGs tell the doctors that Mrs Marsh has a little old heart damage, and a little bit of heart failure, and on examination there was – and the consultant interrupts – 'nothing of serious note'.

So Mrs Marsh's clinical identity is in the process of being transformed: her identity is being shifted, from being someone who is potentially acutely ill, to someone whose underlying problems are chronic and mild. And further, she is being discredited as a witness: she claimed, according to the medical notes, to have *inhaled* a pea. Following the above extract, the consultant goes over to Mrs Marsh and cross-examines her over her signs and symptoms. Through persistently focusing on Mrs Marsh's ankles, how many pillows she uses at night, how far she can walk, the consultant implicates Mrs Marsh's signs and symptoms as due to chronic problems, exacerbated by the current episode, perhaps, but nothing too serious. He does this even in the face of ambiguity raised by Mrs Marsh's responses, such as that she only uses one pillow at night which would normally indicate an absence of heart failure. But then Mrs Marsh as an accurate and reliable witness has already been discredited: she did not choke on a pea, but swallowed a pea. Mrs Marsh also asks a question: she interrupts the consultant's flow and asks when she can go home. This is significant as later on in the ward round the consultant uses her question as an unambiguous expression of Mrs Marsh's desire to go home, and so legitimates his decision to discharge her with an implicit understanding that this is also her choice. After this episode, the consultant and the other members of the ward round go back to the notes trolley and move up the ward well away from Mrs Marsh.

Consultant: (to Lecturer) What are we going to do? I don't want to take her off the tamoxifen – presumably she is on it for a good reason. If we could get her notes and check up on that. And it seems a pity to bronchoscope her. She is in mild heart failure?

Lecturer: She's had frusemide [a diuretic].

Consultant: How much?

Resident: 40.

Consultant: Well, we'll increase that.

Resident: (nods).

Consultant: My feeling would be to let her go home and then bring her back in 10 days to outpatients where either you or Dick could see her. She could have another chest X-ray then. And you could decide if she needs bronchoscopy.

Lecturer: She's got no temperature.

Consultant: She's asymptomatic. [Of what? this is a moment of high ambiguity.] She may have a touch of LVF [left ventricular failure] – with this nocturnal dyspnoea [breathlessness] business. We could send her home on diuretics and you can see her in outpatients in 10 days' time. If it's not all right then you can bronchoscope her. I should think a cooked pea would disintegrate – I should think it would be disintegrating and might just leave a shell. I'll let her out. (to Sister) Sounds as if she would be happy to go home.

Sister: Oh fine – yes.

Consultant: We'll send her home on 80 of frusemide then? (to Resident) And is she on antibiotics?

Resident: No.

Consultant: (to Registrar) And the diagnosis – what would you say – dyspnoea of unknown cause with mild LVF?

Registrar: (nods).

Consultant: (to Senior House Officer) Are you happy with that Geoff?

Senior House   I haven't had anything to do with this lady.
Officer:

Consultant: Oh – I'll just go.

Mrs Marsh's transformation from a patient with a medical future in the unit, to a person who can be discharged is complete: she has breathlessness of *unknown* cause. The consultant has picked up the doubt and the downgrading: Mrs Marsh did not inhale the pea, the pea is not being attributed with the effect, breathlessness, but just in case she did inhale the pea, and it did cause the breathlessness, he would think it would disintegrate. Mrs Marsh's dyspnoea is being implicitly attributed to another narrative: that of the failing heart of an aged woman. The ambiguities are not, however, completely obviated, some uncertainty remains, to be picked up through the outpatients appointment, but importantly the consultant arrives at a 'disposal' (Berg 1992): he reads his colleagues, he reads the patient, he reads the films, he even reads Sister's face. None of these actors appears to be making any objection. But, importantly, what is being staged here is how Mrs Marsh's 'needs' are being *clinically* constituted, through due processes of examination and investigation. And, it is only through these due processes that her needs emerge as not the kinds of needs to be met in an acute medical unit. Any residual need can be taken care of on an outpatient basis.

Sister is consulted once the transformation is almost complete, at the point when the disposal comes into view, for it is she who is charged with the management of the bedstate and with checking a patient's ability and mobility. And Sister had already constituted the patient as ready for discharge *before* the ward round. In her view expressed at the nurses' handover the previous day, Mrs Marsh had nothing of serious note wrong with her, and 'should be ready to go home soon' (field notes). Sister and the doctors are not just transforming Mrs Marsh's identity, they are organising their workplace, as an acute medical ward. They make it possible to reinterpret Mrs Marsh's troubles on other than acute medical grounds, in order to facilitate her disposal, and 'free up' a bed. Any further recovery that Mrs Marsh needs to make can be made at home, where she lives alone but has family and home help involved in her care; thus any remaining needs she may have are constituted as mild, chronic, social and personal. But, critically, the decision is staged as a *clinical one*, to help maintain the purity of the clinical domain.

Discussion

Patients like Mrs Marsh have troubles which are mixtures: she is old and it is her susceptibility to illness which has increased, while her susceptibility to diagnosis and treatment may have decreased. Coupled with these difficulties she has social troubles; she is isolated, with limited resources, she is unproductive, dependent to some degree. Critically then, the doctor manages the diagnosis and treatment of Mrs Marsh in ways which help him dispose of her: she is refigured on the ward round as having, quite simply, no medical future, she has nothing more to be cured. And thus, Mrs Marsh can be discharged because her troubles are inappropriate to an *acute* medical domain.

I want therefore to suggest that 'process-ability' in managerial terms and 'susceptibility' to diagnosis and treatment in medical terms have some kind of congruence, some sort of overlap. Both managerial and medical disciplines work in terms of outcomes and objectives. But what is critical is that for medicine the objective has also been connected to an ethos of care rather than just cost. For medicine there has been a continuous concern with making visible the effectiveness of expertise, underpinned by the notion of progress and movement: this has traditionally included the *diagnosis* of disease, not just the completion of an episode of illness, or the curing of a disease. Most importantly, diagnosis, and sometimes, when lucky, a cure, is shown through the ward round to be accomplished, through the effective (and heroic) application of expertise, in the form of embodied knowledge and skill, 'the medical gaze' (Foucault 1973), *supplemented* by the machines. It is this aspect of traditional medicine which we have seen in the example of Mrs Marsh's ward round. Critically, however, it must be emphasised that she was actually admitted, and there was some care taken over her, because they needed to obtain a diagnosis. Medical practitioners in the past have been much criticised for only being concerned with cure. I want to stress that this is not strictly true: medicine in teaching hospitals such as the one in my example, is also concerned with the practice of diagnosis. And I want to suggest that this is itself an organising principle which has helped maintain the ethos of medicine as concerned, not with social identities but with bodies and their operations. This ethos, under the right conditions, presses doctors to pursue diagnosis even under circumstances which, in the reformation of the health services, may no longer be in their interests. The further erosion of this aspect of medical practice, through introduction of yet more technologies, such as clinical protocols and guidelines which standardise diagnosis may be having unintended consequences, as doctors retreat further and further from the bedside, defending themselves by relocating responsibility for diagnosis with the machines or the guideline, prescribed elsewhere.

Through complex processes of alignment, between the medical and the managerial, it is possible for a continuous, if always failing, purification of the clinical domain through the relentless vigilance of practitioners over the expulsion or exclusion of those patients whose troubles are not susceptible to diagnosis and treatment. The main difficulty is that the complicity between managerial and medical objectives under conditions where there is an erosion of the ethos of care which underpins medicine as a discipline, may be putting patients at risk.

Efficiency has become a hegemony so that good practice is mainly measured in terms of cost, patient throughput and completed consultant episodes, and monitored in terms of accounting technologies. Those patients who are most difficult to diagnose and treat, but who may also be the most needy and vulnerable, such as the very old and the chronically sick may, even during periods of acute illness, be constituted as having troubles which are not reducible to such outcomes, protocols and performance indicators. Thus such patients may be being increasingly excluded from accessing acute medical care. Put simply, their treatment and care is not figured as in doctors', or managers' interests. In the new health services, Mrs Marsh may not even have been admitted, and the precise nature of her 'illness' crosschecked. I do not know if this is a good or bad thing, but it is certainly a vast change in the ethics of health care.

CONCLUSION

The emergence of increasing throughput as a strategic value to help drive health care reforms was not accomplished overnight, nor was it accomplished through coercion, but rather through a subtle arrangement and association of complex and heterogeneous contingent effects. In contrast to other commentators such as Broadbent et al (1991) and many others, these effects themselves can be understood not just as a diffusion (Latimer 1995, Latour 1986) of programmes down through the ranks, nor as the colonisation of the health services by managerialism. Instead, these changes, for their accomplishment, relied upon the enrolment of (some) doctors as members (of a discipline) and, critically, this enrolment was only possible because of a commensurability between the interests of some doctors and the managerial goal of reduction in patients' hospital stays. Indeed, this new emphasis could be understood to be enrolled by doctors in such contexts as the one portrayed, in ways which precisely help them to purify the clinical domain: discourses of efficiency legitimate doctor's disposal of patients who meet neither managerial targets over throughput nor their own, as the production of 'first class medicine' and all that this entails.

For social actors to fall into line so that a set of interests becomes prevalent or dominant, there have to be particular conditions under which these prevailing interests emerge, or appear, as also in their interest. These conditions are not unproblematically put into place, by the introduction of technologies (such as contractual targets), procedures (such as the waiting system) and rules (such as having 10 empty beds each waiting day), although these may certainly be aspects through which particular sets of concerns are made, and kept, present. Rather, in the absence of more direct power effects, such as coercion, the accomplishment of a prevailing set of interests relies on a number of contingent effects, which have to be continuously achieved and re-presented. In this way interests do not lie within individual actors, but between actors, whether human or non-human. Thus interests cannot be taken to only reflect the choices of social actors as individuals, but much, much wider sociocultural relations.

As Latour's example cited earlier emphasises, the subjectivities of social actors must be enrolled if any translation of their interests is to be accomplished. The world is not nearly as functional as the modernists would have it! And it is this feature which I want to pursue in the next chapter in relation to how nurses have been enrolled in issues of increasing throughput and the processing of patients, particularly in relation to how nurses square their conduct to self and others.

REFERENCES

Bachman S, Collard A, Greenberg J, Fountain E, Huebner T, Kimbal B, Melendy K 1987 An innovative approach to geriatric acute care delivery: the Choate-Symmes experience. Hospital and Health Services Administration 32(4): 509–520

Barker W H, Williams T F, Zimmer J G, Van Buren C, Vincent S J, Pickrel S G 1985 Geriatric consultation teams in acute hospitals: impact on back-up of elderly patients. Journal of the American Geriatrics Society 33: 422–428

Berg M 1992 The construction of medical disposals. Medical sociology and medical problem-solving in clinical practice. Sociology of Health and Illness 14(2): 151–180

Bloomfield B, Coombs R, Cooper D J, Rea D 1992 Machines and manoeuvres: responsibility accounting and the construction of hospital information. Accounting, Management and Information Technologies 2(4): 197–219

Bouchier I, Williamson J 1982 The elderly patient in the acute hospital sector. Health Bulletin 40(4): 179–182

Broadbent J, Laughlin R, Read S 1991 Recent financial and administrative changes in the NHS: a critical theory analysis. Critical Perspectives on Accounting 2(1): 1–30

Burley L E, Currie C T, Smith R G, Willliamson J 1979 Contributions of geriatric medicine within acute medical wards. British Medical Journal 2: 90–92

Callon M 1986 Some elements of a sociology of translation: domestication of the scallops and the fishermen of St Brieuc Bay. In: Law J (ed) Power, action and belief: a new sociology of knowledge? Sociological Review Monograph 32. Routledge and Kegan Paul, London, pp 196–233

Clarke J 1996 Public nightmares and communitarian dreams: the crisis of the social in social welfare. In: Edgell S, Hetherington K, Warde A (eds) Consumption matters. Sociological Review Monograph. Blackwell, Oxford

Coid J, Crome P 1986 Bed blocking in Bromley. British Medical Journal 292: 1253–1256

Cooper D J 1988 A social analysis of corporate pollution disclosures: a comment. Advances in Public Interest Accounting 2: 179–186

Currie C T, Smith R G, Williamson J 1979 Medical and nursing needs of elderly patients admitted to acute medical beds. Age and Ageing 8: 149–151

Deetz S 1992 Disciplinary power in the modern corporation. In: Alvesson M, Willmott H (eds) Critical management studies. Sage, London

Department of Health (DoH) 1991 The patient's charter. HMSO, London

Department of Health and Social Security (DHSS) 1981 The respective roles of the general acute and the geriatric sectors in care of the elderly hospital patient. Report of a study. HMSO, London

Dingwall R, Rafferty A M, Webster C 1988 An introduction to the social history of nursing. Routledge, London

Donaldson L J 1983 Care of the elderly in hospitals and homes: foci of discontent. Journal of Rehabilitation and Social Health 5: 181–185

Foucault M 1973 The birth of the clinic. Tavistock, London

Foucault M 1978 Governmentality. In: Burchell G, Gordon C, Miller P (eds) 1991 The Foucault effect. Studies in governmentality. Harvester Wheatsheaf, London

Giddens A 1984 The constitution of society. Outline of structuration theory. Polity Press, Cambridge

Grimley-Evans J 1983 Integration of geriatric with general medical services in Newcastle. Lancet 1: 1430–1433

Hulter Asberg K H 1986 Elderly patients in acute medical wards and home care. Functional assessment, prediction of outcome, and a trial of early activation. PhD Thesis. Comprehensive Summaries of Uppsala Dissertations from the Faculty of Medicine, 25. University of Uppsala, Sweden

Hunter D J 1994 From tribalism to corporatism: the managerial challenge to medical dominance. In: Gabe J, Kelleher D, Williams G (eds) Challenging medicine. Routledge, London

Latimer J 1994 Writing patients, writing nursing: the social construction of nursing assessment of elderly people admitted to an acute medical unit. PhD Thesis, University of Edinburgh

Latimer J 1995 The nursing process re-examined: diffusion or translation? Journal of Advanced Nursing 22: 213–220

Latimer J 1996 Working together. Report of research on collaboration over patient assessment and the organisation of care. Keele University Department of Nursing and Midwifery, Keele

Latimer J 1997 Giving patients a future: the constituting of classes in an acute medical unit. Sociology of Health and Illness 19(2): 160–185

Latimer J 1998 Organising context: nurses' assessments of older people in an acute medical unit. Nursing Inquiry 5(1): 43–57

Latour B 1986 The powers of association. In: Law J (ed) Power, action and belief: a new sociology of knowledge? Sociological Review Monograph 32. Routledge and Kegan Paul, London, pp 264–280

Latour B 1991 Technology is society made durable. In: Law J (ed) A sociology of monsters. Essays on power, technology and domination. Routledge, London

Laughlin R 1996 Principals and higher principals: accounting for accountability in the caring professions. In: Munro R, Mouritsen J (eds) Accountability: power, ethos and the technologies of managing. Thomson International Business Press, London

Loveridge R, Starkey K 1992 Introduction: innovation and interest in the organisation of health care delivery. In: Loveridge R, Starkey K (eds) Continuity and crisis in the NHS. Open University Press, Buckingham

McArdle C, Wylie J C, Alexander W D 1975 Geriatric patients in an acute medical ward. British Medical Journal 4: 568–569

Marcus G, Fischer M 1986 Anthropology as cultural critique: an experimental moment in the human sciences. Chicago University Press, Chicago

Munro R 1992 Enabling participative change: the impact of a strategic value. International Studies in Management and Organization 21(4): 52–65

Munro R 1996 Alignments and identity-work: the study of accounts and accountability. In: Munro R, Mouritsen J (eds) Accountability: power, ethos and the technologies of managing. Thomson International Business Press, London

Rose N, Miller P 1992 Political power beyond the State: problematics of government. British Journal of Sociology 43(2): 173–205

Rubin S G, Davies G H 1975 Bed blocking by elderly patients in general hospital wards. Age and Ageing 4: 142–147

Scottish Hospital Inpatient Statistics. Supplied by the Information and Statistics Division of the Common Services Agency of Scottish Health Services, Edinburgh

Seymour D G, Pringle R 1982 Elderly patients in general surgical units: do they block beds? British Medical Journal 284: 1921–1923

Strong P, Robinson J 1990 The NHS under new management. Open University Press, Milton Keynes

Walton I 1986 The nursing process in perspective. A literature review. Department of Social Policy and Social Work, University of York, York

Interests and identity: nurses conducting care, performing disciplined subjects

8

Joanna Latimer

■ CONTENTS

Introduction 185
Identity and performance: nursing and issues of representation 187
Medicine: constituting the disciplined subject 189
Conducting patient assessment 191
Nursing and the social 194
The constituting of classes 198
Legitimating nursing expertise just by looking 200
Concluding notes on the management of interests and identity 204
References 207

INTRODUCTION

> ... when you start off (nursing) you say 'well I would want to do what the patient would want me to do'. You know, if the patient wants me to sit and blether for half an hour well I would want to sit and blether with them and then you know, but in reality within the constraints of the ward, the ward routine and the set routine and what other people are expecting of you, need from you ... Other patients, medical staff, other learners, and what have you – you tend to end up in a routine and you know, you get somebody up, you give somebody their breakfast, you make somebody's bed, and then you help them to wash, you know, whatever. Wash them whatever it is ... I think you gradually become socialised into the system and nursing. You know, nursing's a routine. ... It, to a certain extent it is, and sometimes I feel very guilty about that and I think 'that's ridiculous, that's terrible', and then at other times *I think 'but we are, this is an acute hospital and you have got to be in a state of readiness, for an emergency, or for a turn of events.*

(Staff Nurse 2, interview, my emphasis)

Interests have emerged in the previous chapter not simply as the bald and barren matter of 'self-interest', the motor of conduct, or coffer of individual credit. Rather, it has been suggested that there is a complex relation between the possibility of enrolling participants, so that they are concerned with, and help accomplish a set of interests, and how this set of interests (seem, at least) to align with, or excite, concerns which are already consistent with some aspects of their identity.

In this chapter I further pursue the complex relations entailed in why practitioners can be enrolled in particular sets of interests. I explore how realignments concern the subjectivities of practitioners, not just as 'individuals', but as participants, or, what Garfinkel (1967) and other ethnomethodologists refer to, as 'members'. Critically, I am suggesting that this complex relation points to how interests are connected to the identity-work of social actors as members of disciplines. I have already suggested that doctors may have been enrolled in aspects of the strategy to increase throughput because they can enrol aspects of this strategy to accomplish the 'discipline' of medicine, as a particular kind of performance. In this chapter I further explore the relation between a translation of interests and identity-work, but this time I focus on nurses.

The chapter begins with discussion of the relationship between identity and performance. Then, drawing on Foucault (1973) I suggest that it is possible to understand that the practice of disciplines, such as medicine, both position and exercise social actors as *subjects*, thus making available a particular subject–knowledge relation for the performance of a disciplinary identity. Using examples from a field study of health care environments concerned with the assessment of acutely ill older people (Latimer 1994, 1997a,b,c, 1998a,b) I show how it is nurses who are concerned with the surveillance of the biographical history of the patient as located in a social and emotional context, and that it is nurses who are the backstage conductors of patient management in relation to their movement through the beds. How they square this conduct with their identities as caring, as well as competent and efficient practitioners, is shown to be complex. An overall effect, it is argued, is that nurses have been more and more enrolled in the organisational politics of acute health care to become conduits for both medical and managerial objectives. However, it is also suggested that this is only possible because it resonates with the complexity and ambivalence present in the identity-work of nursing.

IDENTITY AND PERFORMANCE:
NURSING AND ISSUES OF REPRESENTATION

Contemporary anthropologists and ethnomethodologists have raised the issue of how identity is not something we unproblematically have, such as either our social identity (Joanna is a nurse, she is white, she is middle-aged, she is a mother), or our selfdom. Rather, identity is something connected to issues of representation. Social actors can be represented, and have their identity figured by others (ascribed) but, from a social perspective, identity is something which is ascribed because it is performed. In this sense identity has also to be worked at, or 'performed', continuously. Even a nurse to be ascribed the identity, 'RGN', has to perform in ways to pass (and I mean that in both senses of the term) as an RGN. To hold on to that identity, she must go on passing for a nurse, an RGN, or she risks having her identity questioned or, at worst, being struck off. This is also true of everyday social life: but what constitutes the identity to be passed, and the criteria or marks which will pass, are themselves contested, to be figured and reconfigured locally and specifically.

An individual's identity can be connected to his or her individuality, his or her self. Usually we think of this as *self-identity*. But the identities which we hold out to others, as ourselves, can only be shown through being bodied forth (Strathern 1995) in materials, such as language, and other socially constructed artefacts. Thus these, our selves, are also deeply social because they are only expressible through the deployment of artefacts which are socially and culturally available to us.

Nurses and patients may both be concerned with their identities as individuals, as well as with their identities as kinds of nurses or kinds of person. In the current study I observed nurses and patients as they encountered each other, and I listened to them as they talked with me. Both nurses and patients drew upon culturally available materials to figure themselves and each other, to perform identities which help differentiate them, and qualify their belonging to one category of person rather than another. For example, many of the older people I talked to figured themselves as engaged in active, caring and productive relations. But many of them also appeared to be concerned about the balance of these relations: they were concerned by what they called dependency, and expressed fear at the idea of being any more dependent than they were. Interdependence and reciprocity were, therefore, figured by many of the older people I talked to as of concern to them. Some said that they would rather be dead or put in a home, than be a burden to others. For example, here is an extract from Mr Donald's interview, I have just asked him how he feels about the future:

Mr Donald: In fact the future as far as I'm concerned for over a year, I should be dead, ready laid, right, no regrets, dead! I want to die, I want to die, I want to die!

Researcher: Is that how you're feeling?

Mr Donald: That's how I've felt for over a year, I want to die. Because I've nothing to live for. I'm a man who's never owed other people and I'm having to depend on other people to look after me and I don't want that, I'd rather be dead. See?

Researcher: Really?

Mr Donald: But as far as I'm concerned, now when I get to have my …[?recovery/?discharge], I make the best of it and go home and see how things go. So far, but oh, I would just love something to happen that I could just slip away and be finished with it all.

Mr Donald says he would rather be dead and wishes he might just slip away. In his account he is presenting himself as someone who is not normally dependent upon others: he was a man who never owed anybody. But he does not leave the matter there, he would lose face as miserable and ungrateful. He offers another face: he's resigned to make the best of a bad job and just 'see how things go'. Dependency and becoming a burden characterise a portentous leitmotif found in many of the patients' discourses; through it they were figuring themselves as, for example, *responsible* persons. Interests and concerns, therefore, can be expressive of identity, they can help mark someone as belonging to one kind of group rather than another kind of group, or as one kind of person rather than another. Usually of course, it is configurations of different features which make up identity.

Importantly, identity is connected to 'kinds': categories and classes of things. But there are marks which will pass for some kinds of things rather than other kinds of things. For example, a professional identity is distinguished by certain characteristics, such as a particular degree of intelligence, altruism, or intuition, or a manner of conduct. Critically, professionals have knowledge and skills which others do not have, but which have to be acquired through educational and other practices. But it is not enough to have these things, they must be performed and displayed, continuously. Critically, the marks that will pass for a professional identity are both contestable and are deployed in the management of interests.

MEDICINE:
CONSTITUTING THE DISCIPLINED SUBJECT

The performance of medicine for its disciplinary power relies upon how it makes the invisible (disease processes, their origins and causes) visible and, thereby, knowable. Foucault (1973) gives clinical medicine a fundamental place in what he calls the 'architecture of the human sciences' (p. 198). It is fundamental because it is a discourse founded on 'positive knowledge'; that is, knowledge derived from actual observation and experience of the body and its pathologies as natural phenomena, rather than of disease as a 'metaphysics of evil' (p. 196):

> illness, counter-nature, death, in short, the whole dark underside of disease came to light, at the same time illuminating and eliminating itself like night, in the deep, visible, solid, enclosed, but accessible space of the human body. What was fundamentally invisible is suddenly offered to the brightness of the gaze, in a movement of appearance so simple, so immediate that it seems to be the natural consequence of a more highly developed experience.
>
> (Foucault 1973, p. 195)

Foucault is suggesting that medicine's methods set it apart as a new form of science. Its methods included making the body accessible and visible through cutting it up, classifying and categorising its traits and parts, mapping out its structures and operations, directly observing the manifestations of disease, allowing them to run their natural course. So that (discursively) medicine claims to know disease by seeing it, and through categorising its signs and symptoms, medicine built a body of knowledge, which can be learnt and passed on. This was the new myth, that man could know by seeing, but, crucially, with an informed or *disciplined* gaze. Medicine thus emerges as instituting a positivism which continues to penetrate all human sciences and our belief in them today. It attempted to (and this remains at the heart of medical ideology) 'free itself of theories and chimeras, to approach the object of their (clinical doctors') experience with the purity of an unprejudiced gaze' (Foucault 1973, p. 195). In these ways, the discipline of medicine exercises the subject (the doctor) as both a knowing subject *and* as an ethical (unprejudiced) subject.

Central to the formation of a new order of knowledge is the abstraction of the doctor in relation to the patient as a social being: 'In order to know the truth of the pathological fact, the doctor must abstract the patient.' (Foucault 1973, p. 8).

Thus the particulars of the patient, his social details, were transformed into phenomena which were likely to get in the way of understanding the disease. Rather, medicine laid claims to establishing its positive knowledge by appearing to free knowledge about the body and disease from emotion, superstition and metaphysics, through basing its methods on observation, that is on direct experience of the real world, through seeing with a pure uncluttered gaze and by making the invisible visible. The transformatory power of this discourse in our ontology lies in this displacement of things: medicine changes the order of things and seeks to transform the social to construct a neutral, disciplined space.

The subject–object divide is constituted through the practice of examination. Through subjectification of the patient under examination, the examiner constitutes the patient as an object and himself as the subject who is objective. The subject (doctor) is '*looking* according to a grid of perceptions' and '*noting* according to a code' (Foucault 1991, p. 56), and it is in this way that the doctor, as disciplined subject, can displace the social aspects of his experience, the subject 'listening, interpreting, deciphering' (Foucault 1991, p. 56). The gaze defines the *space* in which things can be thought of, so that they are seen/noticed. In this way the subject himself (the doctor) exercises and is exercised through the gaze. This in turns performs his disciplined identity. In these ways, forms of social distance can be affected through his perspectival seeing: through the gaze, he constitutes any encounter with the other as concerned with particulars, as predecided by the discourse which he draws upon to constitute his gaze. The other, with his concerns and perspectives and beliefs, can be displaced.

The setting under study, an acute medical unit in a prestigious UK teaching hospital, was, according to the Professor of Medicine who headed up the unit, concerned with the practice of first class medicine. The ward round concerning Mrs Marsh, discussed in the previous chapter, is an example of such a practice as a particular process of examination and diagnosis. However, as we have already noted, the practice of first class medicine relies to some extent on processes of exclusion of patients who do not have resolvable problems. Differentiating such patients, however, relies on an extension of the medical gaze to those very domains of social life which are potentially polluting to medicine, because they involve reintroducing the patient as a social being.

CONDUCTING PATIENT ASSESSMENT

In the field study described in the introduction to the book, and in the previous chapter, it emerges in the discourses of practitioners that the hospital did not just diagnose and cure sick bodies. Practitioners also talked about and were concerned with 'beds', 'admissions' and 'discharges'. In this way practitioners were as involved in the performance of the discipline of medicine as they were in a distribution of resources.

Importantly, the use of the term 'beds', qualified by their availability status, was also metaphoric: it helped signify movement, movement through the hospital, the flow. Arrangements for the admission of acutely ill patients to the 'main' hospital, to gaining access to a bed, have deep meanings for staff. They were associated with making sure the right sorts of patients get admitted to the right kinds of beds. But establishing what constitutes the right kinds of patients is extremely complex. It relies upon much more than the application of the pure and unadulterated medical gaze, as exemplified in a conversation I had with several qualified nurses soon after I commenced the study.

The context of the conversation was the introduction of an overnight admissions ward. I asked Sister what she thought the rationale was for this organisational change. She and two of the Staff Nurses were standing around the nurses' station, checking medicines and equipment:

Sister: It's to stop the wards being disturbed at night.

Senior Staff Nurse:	It's also so that some patients can be discharged straight home if necessary. They need a geriatrician on the admissions unit. A lot of patients are geriatric and should never get to the medical wards.
Sister:	They're admitted because they've fallen at home and they need mobilising and rehabilitation, physiotherapy and occupational therapy. But they're admitted here and they're here for weeks. They don't have any medical problems.
Researcher:	So what is a 'geriatric' patient.
Sister:	Elderly.
Senior Staff Nurse:	Frail, old, gone off their legs a bit.
Second Staff Nurse:	(who had been listening while at the drug trolley) Ward 10 [the geriatric assessment ward in the hospital] is always half empty and they're admitted here because they won't take acute admissions to the ward there, only referrals.

The nurses explain the opening of the admission ward in terms of stopping the wards from being disturbed at night, and in terms of a gate-keeping function: it is a way of stopping unnecessary admissions. This leads on to their discussing how there are inappropriately placed people in their ward. They construct a category of patient who is inappropriate: geriatrics. To do this nurses bring into play systems of distinction: geriatrics 'fall', they are 'frail, old, gone off their legs'. But, importantly, geriatrics are also being distinguished, not because they have no needs, but as having needs which are inappropriate to the unit. To constitute geriatrics as different, the nurses mobilise aspects of discourse on geriatric nursing/medicine: 'geriatrics' require 'mobilising and rehabilitation, physiotherapy and occupational therapy', not acute medical care. Their needs are functional, rather than bio-physiological. So some patients, then, are constituted, not as 'well', but as having needs which are not related to diagnosis and cure.

Critically, nurses, in their assessments, do not just identify a need (falling, incontinence, etc.) but qualify the nature of a need in relation to its cause. It is the attribution of causality, or the grounds upon which a need can be explained, that qualify the nature of the need to figure the identity of the patient. For example, in the following extract the same Staff Nurse and Sister went on to talk about a patient who is in the category of 'long-term geriatric' to exemplify their point:

Sister: Take Jessie. She came to us as a purely social admission. She'd fallen at home and is incontinent. She had turned against her home help, refused to answer the door to let her in. She didn't become 91 overnight, she's been old for a long time. She had been going downhill. She's been here ever since. She didn't have any medical problems. What is the GP doing, is what I would like to know. She should have been on the long-term waiting list and assessed by the GP, and admitted there. Not here.

Researcher: So why did she come in?

Sister: She had fallen. She is incontinent.

Researcher: What about the stroke? [Jessie's 'diagnosis' at report is cerebrovascular accident – CVA.]

Staff Nurse: Oh she had that after she came in. She's gone downhill. She used to walk with a Zimmer [a walking frame] and dress and wash herself. That's how she managed at home. Now she needs long-term care.

Sister: She is purely a social problem.

Researcher: So why did she fall?

Staff Nurse: She had gone off her legs a bit, frail, you know, old and frail.

The nurses are aligning many heterogeneous materials to construct their assessment of Jessie: for example, her falls and her incontinence, her non-compliant conduct, her age, the management of her care in the community. Sister states categorically that she did not have any medical problems. The nurses configure Jessie in ways to show that her needs are the natural consequence of old age, and a steady decline to death. Even when reminded of Jessie's stroke, the Staff Nurse refigures the stroke as a natural, not a medical phenomenon, and that Jessie's consequent needs are social, not medical.

These nurses are charged with, and in their talk and interviews with me, pride themselves upon their contribution to the care and diagnosis of the acutely ill medical patient, but if that is all they were, the doctors' eyes in their absence, they would not be distinguishing themselves as different. Constituting themselves as caring and therefore different is not an available discourse: as Davies (1995) has explicated, caring is dichotomised from professional competence in the logic of health care organisation. Rather, nurses can be distinctive because they are competent in relation to more than just their contribution to the diagnosis and medical treatment of a patients' troubles: they are competent in relation to their contribution to helping maintain the flow of patients through the beds. The work of maintaining the flow relies upon bringing the social into the medical domain but at the same time as it is held apart from, and remains constituted as supplementary* to, the pure work of diagnosis and cure.

NURSING AND THE SOCIAL

The ethos of nursing figured in nursing discourse characterises nurses, and distinguishes nurses from doctors, because they are concerned with the impact of disruptions to health upon the functional and psychosocial lives of patients as unique individuals. It is this aspect of nurses' performances in the current context which allow their alignment with arrangements for increasing throughput: performing patient assessment over the psychosocial and functional aspects of a patient's situation helps nurses to demonstrate a distinctive identity from doctors, as at the same time it helps accomplish a concern for patients as made up of more than their bio-physiological status. Nurses' accounts are now drawn on to elaborate this relation.

The nurses in the current study referred to how they need to know about a patient's 'social situation'. Other ways of referring to this area of concern were 'home-life', 'context' and 'lifestyle'. These matters were associated for the nurses with 'mobility', 'self-care' ability and 'support'.† Taken together these matters for some of the nurses were

---

* I am drawing on an idea of Strathern's (1997). For Strathern Euro-American relations, such as the male–female relation, are ordered by processes of contrasting identities (comparison), one of which must always be supplementary to the other, rather than through differences which are complementary.

† These accounts must not be confused with nurses presenting themselves as in social relations with their patients, through which they know what patients need. Nurses help maintain the supplementary nature of the social to the medical, through referring to a social life as something patients need, but which they, the nurses, did not have time for. In contrast, the surveillance of the social life of patients is incorporated as significant to the techniques of nurses' knowledge practices.

wrapped in the concept 'capability' and its opposite, 'disability'. The nurses claimed that it is important to know what a patient's 'home' or 'social' situation is like: this concept is evolved in their accounts in relation to notions of family support, usual 'self-care' ability, mobility, and about any social services involved. These features act together to indicate how capable a patient is, normally or prior to the current episode of illness.

Sister claimed that knowing about a patient's normal mobility or self-care ability enables comparison to know what is abnormal in the present situation:

Sister: We always get a history from a patient or from the relatives to see what they were like prior to admission. And if they were mobile prior to admission you think why aren't they mobile now?

In this extract Sister associates the 'admitting' process with getting a 'history' of a patient. Getting a 'history' has a specific purpose – to alert Sister to discrepancies, particularly in mobility, and to 'see' what a patient 'was like' prior to admission. What Sister looks for are 'signs', this is apparent in her response to a question asking when it was difficult to get information:

Sister: Yes. We found, I find it difficult when an elderly lady has come in and confused having been found collapsed and not coping at home. Can't give us any kind of history as to what's wrong with her, and we find that she has never had any help whatsoever and she has no family. And it's very, very difficult. Very often they don't want to accept any social help that's the problem with them. So generally we have to send the OT [occupational therapist] off to their home, get involved with the social worker and then go off and look round the home to decide how suitable or unsuitable it is.

So normally a history enables Sister to make an assessment of patients in terms of their social situation and their capability. But here, no history from the patient acts in combination with something in the presenting problems to alert Sister of the need to obtain more information about a patient's home and her history.

In giving an example where apparent breakdown in an older person's life leads to having to send out into the community to 'look' for further evidence of this person's life, Sister is giving some indication as to how she normally tells or judges a person's social situation. 'Confused', 'collapsed', 'no help whatsoever', 'no family', 'found not coping at home'. These act as traces for Sister: they act in combination to signify something about this person's life in relation to her ability to be at home. In the above extreme case she is alerted to a situation which is 'very, very difficult'.

It would seem from Sister's talk that she differentiates how much you need to know about a person on the basis of the particular set of conditions: the person's social situation and past have significance in particular situations. In talking about what information she needs to know about patients generally, Sister did not raise the issue of a patient's past or home life, except in relation to the elderly and the chronically disabled:

Sister: I think it is very important especially with a view to them going back. If they've come in having collapsed at home and are unable to cope at home you don't want to send them back into the same situation without any help, for them to bounce back into hospital within 2 or 3 days. You need to know whether they've got home helps, meals on wheels, district nurse, hospital club or day hospitals or social clubs that they go to. Usually if their relatives are staying with them, are their relatives prepared to look after them for a little while after they come out of hospital or are the relatives prepared to put a bit more input into them when they are discharged? You need to know quite a lot about a patient, you need to know whether they live upstairs in a flat, you need to know whether they're on a ground floor or ...

Sister is emphasising how it is important to know about a patient's social situation and his or her family life 'with a view to them going back'. There is no sense of how it can impact on the present, in relation to understanding the nursing requirements of a patient who is in hospital with an acute illness. Sister envisages 'social situation' in terms of support to enable 'coping', and relates this to discharge arrangements, matters which are specifically important in relation to older patients. The implication is that older people may be in hospital because of their situation: 'you don't want to send them home into the same situation without any help, for them to bounce back into hospital'.

From her talk it would appear that Sister only regards a patient's past as important where there is a potential or actual problem in his or her 'social situation', specifically in terms of the patient's 'capability', that is mobility and 'self-care' ability, and how this is balanced against the support the patient needs and can get. There were two groups of patients whose past she was interested in: the elderly and at another point she also mentions the chronically ill. In the case of younger patients she assumes them to be normally fit; the past, and their home life have no particular significance:

Sister: You certainly wouldn't ask a 19-year-old who's come in having had a query pneumonia if they have a home-help or district nurse or health visitor or, that's a different kind of, well, because you assume before they came in they were quite able to look after themselves. But the elderly on the other hand they do need a lot of social support.

So some patients' past conduct or social support is irrelevant because you 'assume' that they are able to look after themselves and, most importantly, they do not need any extra support in the future to enable them to get home. This helps to clarify how these matters are not in anyway being constituted as important to the practice of medical diagnosis and treatment. The social and the medical are continuously held apart. And through the nature of the association of the social with older people, with people who may have no medical *or* social future, the social is simultaneously and continuously being downgraded, as supplementary to the medical.

Staff Nurse 3 talks in terms of 'phases' of illness: once the acute phase of illness is over, mobilisation begins, and it is in relation to this aspect that knowing about the 'past' is important, because it enables you to judge the future. She says, 'We have a vague idea of how good they are anyway, so we know what to aim for, so we know what we're trying to get them to do.' Patients' 'mobility', their ability to cope normally and their 'goodness' are interrelated in some way: knowing what their 'best' is gives something to aim for, something to get back to.

As can be seen, the nurses mentioned the importance of knowing about the patient's 'past' in terms of specific concepts relating to a patient's ability to cope or self-care. What emerges is that this is particularly important in relation to a patient's future – a patient's potential for discharge, or his or her 'disposability'. But knowing what someone was like normally, some of the nurses claimed, also gives something to aim for in the rehabilitation of patients. For Sister this is an important aspect as it gives you a 'goal'. Similarly for Staff Nurse 3 an important aspect of knowing how people are usually in terms of their 'capability' is that it gives you something realistic to aim for because it helps *classify* them.

THE CONSTITUTING OF CLASSES

In the following extract, Staff Nurse 4 is talking about a patient she admitted the day before who had been described by the doctor in A&E (accident and emergency) as a 'total wreck' with a 'knackered heart':

Staff Nurse 4: … so in that case we were able to see she was capable of quite a lot … so already we could assess that she was capable of doing a lot for herself. So I spoke to the patient, I spoke to her daughter, and, em, I got a clear picture in my mind and then wrote up the care plan according to what I thought her needs were from there.

Researcher: … So what sort of things did you get from them?

Staff Nurse 4: Basically a history of what has happened over the past few days, for a start, leading up to the admission, so the recent history as to what led up to the admission. A history of what she was like before she took ill this time, so that at least for long-term means you know how good you're trying to get the patient back to.

Researcher: You got a base to …?

Staff Nurse 4: You've got a baseline picture. Now, I know that up until Sunday this woman was em, totally self-caring, so if we were thinking now in the long term we're trying to get this patient back to that, to that level. So up until Sunday she was totally looking after herself.

Staff Nurse 4 stresses how knowing about the patient in the past in terms of her capability acts as a 'baseline picture'. It is very important in terms of being able to aim for something: her metaphor, 'baseline' and 'level', implies that the past acts as an objective measurement by which to judge the patient's rehabilitation. It also implies some sort of scale. There is also the implication that Staff Nurse 4 is going to nurse the patient in the present in a different way because she knows that 'up until Sunday this woman was, em, totally self-caring'; she was 'totally looking after herself'.[‡] Staff Nurse 4 stresses this aspect of the patient's history in a way which implies that she is going to nurse this woman in a way which is appropriate to someone who is normally self-caring, rather than nurse her as someone who has been totally dependent for some time.

Staff Nurse 4 is classifying the patient in a similar way to Staff Nurse 3, who stated that the past gives you something realistic to aim for. For Staff Nurse 4, the past gives her an idea of 'how good you're trying to get'.

Patients are classified by nurses partly in relation to a scale of goodness, which is associated with their level of capability. The discourses about Jessie, discussed earlier, constitute Jessie as not just capable of very little, but as obstructive and as not wanting to help herself at all. As an effect of this she is constituted as a class of patient who is inappropriate to the acute medical domain, she is merely social, and has no medical future. In contrast, Staff Nurse 4 *sees* (with her own eyes) her patient as capable of quite a lot, and supplements what she sees with what she hears: that her patient was totally self-caring up until Sunday. She is then able to move her patient up the scale, to reclassify her as having a medical future.

Nurses' concerns, then, for taking into account aspects of the social and functional aspects of patients' lives are perhaps *passable* in an acute care context where there is emphasis on throughput, but also it should be noted nurses are themselves enrolling the notion that

---

[‡] I should mention at this point that throughout the study the notion of self-care, and the will to self-care, was constituted as one aspect of a positive identity by which to classify patients, and amounted to what Rudge has called a nursing hegemony (Rudge 1997). As an aspect of how persons are categorised, or categorise themselves, self-care as a measure of a patient's capability and worth it is consistent with patients' fears of a loss of identity through becoming more and more dependent, mentioned earlier in relation to Mr Donald's account through which he figures himself as preferring death to increased dependency.

knowing about these aspects of patients is critical to generating their mobility and maintaining the flow through the beds. Thus, nurses are enrolled in and are enrolling an interest in throughput in their talk about how their assessment practices and concerns over patients extend far beyond a patient's bio-physiological function. But they are also doing more identity-work than this: they are performing themselves as concerned with notions of progress and heroism accomplished through their own ways of knowing as disciplined subjects.

LEGITIMATING NURSING EXPERTISE
JUST BY LOOKING

In their interviews with me nurses talked about getting to know about patients in terms of what was *visible*. 'Looking' at patients should be understood as having both a literal and virtual meaning for the nurses. There was in their talk constant reference to knowing aspects of patients' requirements in terms of 'seeing', 'looking', 'getting a picture'. While it is recognised here that in everyday language 'seeing' and 'looking' are used as dead metaphors, in the present context 'looking' as method for the nurses had a deeper significance.

Staff Nurse 1 says that her initial way of finding out about how a patient is would be to 'look at her'. She said that she could tell 'just by looking at them if they're in pain', but that she would then cross-check by asking – ' You know, how are you?' She also claimed that on doctors' ward rounds, she could 'tell just by looking at the patient if they're confused by what they've [the doctors] said, if they're anxious or whatever', so that she would know to return to the patient afterwards and help elucidate what the doctors have said. This nurse is claiming that she can understand some of the patients' requirements, some of what is going on in the inside, by reading their behaviour through looking. She is prepared to cross-check her reading of the situation through talk with the patient, but the emphasis for her was on seeing for herself and reading what she sees as the visible signs of the patient's experience. In her examples, 'pain' and 'confusion' are manifest in behaviour, made visible through application of the expert nursing gaze which can read behaviour as signs.

A further aspect of the nurses' 'look' is appraisal of the patient: summing up how the patient is. In the following extract, Staff Nurse 3 is talking about how she knows what people need from her:

> Staff Nurse 3: Well I think a lot of people you can just assess very quickly when they come in, just by the way they act. Usually it's easy to spot if someone's really anxious when they do first come in ...

Staff Nurse 3 is making the claim that she can assess 'a lot of people' quickly when they come in 'just by the way they act'. For example, knowing that patients are anxious can be seen by the way they act, it is easy to 'spot'. For this nurse, knowing whether or not a patient is anxious is important because she believes that some people can get into 'such a state that they can actually exacerbate their illness'. She says that when a patient has chest pain and is really anxious you would then need to 'keep a special eye on them', perhaps use talk to help the patient get through it.

Staff Nurse 3 does not discuss anxiety in terms of talk and a patient's voice resonance, but in terms of a way of seeing, which is in some way informed and judgemental, in the sense of making a judgement. The expression 'act' here may refer to the observable manifestations of anxiety in a patient's behaviour, such as the arrangement of the face and hands, his or her eye movements, what is called 'body language'. The expression 'act' may also include the speech dimension, so-called speech-acts. But Staff Nurse 3 is describing her method of knowing only in terms of seeing, 'spot', in terms of what is visible.

Staff Nurse 3 goes on to contrast this immediate way of knowing about patients by 'spotting', with situations where patients are in some way not themselves, not able to act themselves, that is when they are 'confused' or 'clapped out'. In this instance, Staff Nurse 3 claims, 'you' ask someone else who knows the patient, what they are 'usually like'. Staff Nurse 3 is saying that it is important to know how a patient is 'usually' but that certain conditions dis-enable patients from 'act'-ing as they 'usually' are; she cannot then 'see' them 'act' how they are. In this situation she claims that she gets to know about how they 'usually' are through talk. But talk in her mind is converted or translated into an image, into the visible: she uses talk to help 'build' up a 'picture' of someone over time. Although this phrase is resonant with the phrase 'the mind's eye', it implies translating what becomes known, through talking with relatives, into thinking as if it has been observed, thinking talk as visible. So, for Staff Nurse 3, even what goes on on the inside of people – their feelings and experience of the present – is somehow observable, knowable by seeing.

Staff Nurse 2 talks about 'looking' for herself when she was worried about a particular aspect of a patient's condition she wanted to be 'observed', such as pressure areas. Seeing for herself here is related to 'knowing for sure'. This nurse felt that only by seeing for herself could she be sure of something. She also discussed how 'looking' on the morning drug round enabled her to do a crude assessment of how patients were:

Staff Nurse 2:   Oh well it's just a general, I mean anybody who say is looking very breathless or is looking as though they are in pain, or is looking, it's just basic crude observations you know, that you've a person with a left ventricular [failure] and you've just been told their weight's up and you notice they're sitting gasping for breath, you think 'I'll get something done about this, see about you later'. Just very crude, not all the ins and outs of how, what they've been thinking about overnight, just a crude assessment.

Staff Nurse 2 is inverting 'looking': she gives 'looking' (like something) to the patient, so that she can 'observe' their problem. She announces that this is 'just basic crude observations', and contrasts it with what presumably she thinks of as less crude assessment: 'all the ins and outs, what they've been thinking about overnight'.

For this Staff Nurse there are aspects of assessment which are visible and relate to signs which correspond to certain problems a patient can have, like pain or breathlessness, aspects which she can 'get something done about' or 'see about … later'. From what she says later in the interview she is referring here to informing the doctor about the patient. She implies that previous information given to her, relating to the patient's diagnosis and current 'condition' ('left ventricular failure' and 'their weight is up') directs or gives meaning to what she is seeing, transforming into the technical, her 'observation'. Medical discourse makes visible what she is looking at: a patient 'gasping for breath' contains both *auditory* ('gasping' as sound of 'laboured intake of breath') and *visual* ('gasping' as 'mouth gaping open with chest heaving up and down') information about a patient. Staff Nurse 3 transforms both into visible evidence, 'observations', which supports what she has been told in terms of the so-called facts about the patient, that the patient has heart failure and that his weight is up. (Staff Nurse 5 explains how they observe fluid intake and output and weigh all patients on diuretics, which usually signifies some sort of heart failure, so that they daily can 'see' if the patient is 'actually passing urine'.)

Staff Nurse 4 talks about 'telling' how a patient is by giving 'the patient the once-over', and 'just looking at their overall state'. The 'once-over' has the sense of a quick appraisal, a look which takes in the patient from head to toe: in conjunction with the notion of 'looking' the sense is of the patient as the object of the nurse's experienced gaze, from which she can read the signs, understand signs which serve to disclose not just the body's secrets but also the mind's. As Staff Nurse 4 says 'just really by looking at a patient you can tell how they really are'. The more experienced you are the easier this becomes.

What Staff Nurse 4 describes is an informed way of seeing which takes as its central focus the patient's activity in relation to medical discourse. For example, she describes her admission of a patient that she refers to as the woman with the 'knackered heart'. She says that she could see that the patient was able to support herself and that she was not 'collapsed', the colour of her skin indicated her breathing and circulation were able to suffuse her body adequately (in the staff nurse's view), she was able to get off the trolley on to the bed unaided, she was able to 'give a history' presumably, in Staff Nurse 4's opinion, by answering questions lucidly without compromising her breathing, giving further evidence of adequate circulation, especially to the brain. So 'we were able to see she was capable of quite a lot'. Here capability is made *visible* through translation of signs of activity by the cipher of the nurses' discourse.

The translation is made possible by an understanding of the meaning of the signs in the ordered world of the medical discourse on the body's circulation. 'So then we've moved up, up my scale from total chaos': Staff Nurse 4's metaphor would indicate that she believes that, at some level, her ability to 'see' a patient's capability is analogous to a measuring instrument. A 'clear picture in my mind' came after talk, with the patient and with her daughter; the auditory gave clarity to what she had seen, which was in conflict with what she had been told. From this, the Staff Nurse says that she was able to construct a care plan; that is, make decisions about the patient's nursing care requirements.

It should be emphasised how 'clinical' the nurse's assessment is: she presents herself as a cognitive subject (she does not mention feelings or intuition), she speaks about herself as looking and as deciding for herself. But as has already been indicated, the central point of reference is not how the patient is feeling, her comfort and the relief of her suffering, but how capable the patient is. The gaze is searching to estimate the patient's value in relation to the good of getting her mobile again, as opposed to the evil of someone who is immovable: 'So then we've moved up, up my scale from total chaos'.

Nurses, in the current study, are caught in a web of concerns: on the one hand, they have a need to show that their practices are effective and competent because they are disciplined, so that they are considered as more than just intuitive or female carers, but on the other they are caught in the supplementary relation of the social to the medical.

CONCLUDING NOTES ON THE MANAGEMENT OF INTERESTS AND IDENTITY

In the previous chapter I have discussed how medical[§] participants in acute health care contexts have been enrolled in, and enrol, the strategic value of increasing throughput, augmented through health care reforms during the 1980s. More recent reforms have attempted to make more and more explicit the relation between throughput, cost containment and the performance targets of individual doctors and trusts. The focus on patient throughput has therefore become a *dominant* value and, because it resonates with some aspects of the performance of acute medicine, it has had several crucial effects, which were or were not intended (for discussion of unintended consequences, see Giddens 1984). Indeed it is the unintended consequences of policy agendas which are of interest here: it is the process of mapping and pointing to these effects which undermines any notion

---

[§] I am very unhappy with this distinction: I consider many participants as engaged in a distributed medical practice, not just doctors, but the term doctors is immediately individualising, which is itself something which I would prefer to avoid.

that we can (or indeed should want to) control and predict the action of policy in practice.

One effect is that medicine is not just being managed, but is increasingly charged with managing patients, so that medicine can now be qualified as 'managing'. Another effect has been, where a patient's movement through the beds and out of the hospital may be called into doubt, as in the case of older people, practitioners focus as much on their potential mobility, and discharge, as their diagnosis and cure. This may or may not have had some positive consequences, such as that practitioners may be alert to the need to have in mind and be partially responsible for patients' post-admission needs, a notoriously problematic area for most hospital practitioners. But it has had a further effect.

I want to suggest that enrolling doctors in acute care contexts in managing (and processing) patients is intimately connected to the *purpose* of health care systems and the division of labour. Rather than defining health as concerned with functional, social and experiential as well as bio-physiological issues, strategies over increasing throughput have made the division between what are health issues which are of concern to acute health care professionals, and health issues which are of concern to others, such as patients themselves, or primary care practitioners, or lay carers, more explicit. Indeed, an increase in throughput does not just rely upon the more efficient use of hospital resources (i.e. beds, clinic appointments, investigations and tests, examination and assessment, and other resources), it relies upon an increasingly explicit *division* between the medical and the social aspects of health and illness. Ironically, in the case of older people as discussed in the previous chapter, the efficient management of their care is also seen to rely on the incorporation of a review of their illness in relation to aspects of their social, emotional and functional situation.

Some would say that this shift has resulted in more and more responsibility for health and care being shifted onto patients themselves, and onto the family, particularly women (see, for example, Gregor 1997). I am suggesting, however, that enrolling notions of increasing throughput helps medical practitioners in acute care contexts justify exclusion (or expulsion) of those very patients whose troubles can be shown to be chronic, the effects of time or age, and in need of social rather than medical solutions. It is possible, then, that doctors have been enrolled in managerial agendas concerned with increasing throughput because they can enrol these agendas to help them in their continuous attempt to purify the acute medical domain of 'normal rubbish' (see Jeffrey 1979). This is not because doctors are self-interested and calculating individuals (although some of them may be!), rather, some patients get constituted in these ways because, as I have already suggested in the previous chapter, they present difficulties for the practise of medicine under conditions where the patient may not be susceptible to a progressive and heroic model of diagnosis and cure. This is not just a functional concern, but is also a critical aspect of medicine as an ethical practice, from which, as I have suggested in the previous chapter, many benefits may or may not accrue to the public good.

At first sight (or thought) it is much more difficult to understand the alignment of nurses with the moves to increase throughput, because it appears, for nurses at least, to clash with their professional concerns in relation to the comprehensive care of patients as individuals. But under conditions where nurses are increasingly made accountable for their practices, and where what has accountability is restricted to what can be made visible as purposeful work (see also Walton 1986, Latimer 1999), justifying caring for patients with little 'prospect ahead of them' (Staff Nurse, field notes) emerges as deeply problematic. But, as I have shown, determining whether patients have a prospect ahead of them, relies on a particular kind of assessment, an assessment which entails the surveillance of the patients' social situation, their biography and recent history, their capability and their willingness to mobilise. In other words, the very aspects of patient assessment which were made absent from the ward round in the previous chapter, because they must be kept supplementary to the spectacle of the important and primary work of the setting, that is the diagnosis (and, sometimes, the cure) of disease, are the review of the patient's functional and social situation. They are only present in the form of Sister's agreement, for it is the nurses who are charged with these aspects of patient care.

Nurses legitimate their practices in relation to how a patient moves, from 'chaos, up, up the scale'. Nurses, to show that they have competence, that they have a purpose, must show that they have outcomes. Only some patients will do: like the doctors, nurses need patients who can help them make a showing. Patients like Jessie do not move, they are heavy on other acutely ill patients, heavy on the wards, heavy on staff. In the hands of nurses in the current context, nursing discourse, embodied in the nursing process, gets translated: what gets left out is the notion that the patients themselves can participate in the identification of their needs or wants, or that the patient is an experiencing subject who needs to be taken account of. This is relegated as social. As the Staff Nurse puts it, in the passage quoted at the beginning of this chapter:

> ... sometimes I feel very guilty about that and I think 'that's ridiculous, that's terrible', and then at other times *I think 'but we are, this is an acute hospital and you have got to be in a state of readiness, for an emergency, or for a turn of events'.*
>
> (Staff Nurse 2, interview, my emphasis)

REFERENCES

Davies C 1995 Gender and the professional predicament in nursing. Open University Press, Buckingham

Foucault M 1973 The birth of the clinic. Tavistock, London

Foucault M 1991 Politics and the study of discourse. In: Burchell, Gordon, Miller (eds) The Foucault effect: studies in governmentality. Harvester Wheatsheaf, London

Garfinkel H 1967 Studies in ethnomethodology. Prentice-Hall, Englewood Cliffs, New Jersey

Giddens A 1984 The constitution of society. Outline of structuration theory. Polity Press, Cambridge

Gregor F 1997 From women to women: nurses, informal caregivers and the gender dimension of health care reform. Health and Social Care in the Community 5(1): 30–36

Jeffrey R 1979 Normal rubbish: deviant patients in casualty departments. Sociology of Health and Illness 1(1): 91–107

Latimer J 1994 Writing patients, writing nursing: the social construction of nursing assessment of elderly people admitted to an acute medical unit. PhD Thesis, University of Edinburgh

Latimer J 1997a Giving patients a future: the constituting of classes in an acute medical unit. Sociology of Health and Illness 19(2): 160–185

Latimer J 1997b Older people in hospital: the labour of division, affirmation and the stop. In: Hetherington K, Munro R (eds) Ideas of difference: social spaces and the labour of division. Sociological Review Monograph. Blackwells, Oxford, pp 273–297

Latimer J 1997c Figuring identities: older people, medicine and time. In: Jamieson A, Harper S, Victor C (eds) Critical approaches to ageing and later life. Open University Press, Milton Keynes, pp 143–159

Latimer J 1998 Organising context: nurses' assessments of older people in an acute medical unit. Nursing Inquiry 5(1): 43–57

Latimer J 1999 The dark at the bottom of the stair: participation and performance of older people in hospital. Medical Anthropology Quarterly 13(2)

Rudge T 1997 Nursing wounds: a discourse analysis of nurse–patient interactions during wound care procedures in a burns unit. PhD Thesis, La Trobe University, Melbourne, Australia

Strathern M 1995 The relation. Issues in complexity and scale. Prickly Pear Press, Cambridge

Strathern M 1997 Gender: division or comparison? In: Hetherington K, Munro R (eds) Ideas of difference: social spaces and the labour of division. Sociological Review Monograph. Blackwells, Oxford pp 42–63

Walton I 1986 The nursing process in perspective. A literature review. Department of Social Policy and Social Work, University of York, York

Epilogue

In this book we have together stated our commitment to an intellectual critique of some aspects of contemporary health care. The *competing interests* of the subtitle have been brought out in our analysis of the policies underpinning health care practice and the different possibilities for the distribution of health care as an important social resource. What we have shown is how defining health need and prioritising its distribution is complex and open to competing interests and interpretations.

Although an historical chronology was never intended, the discussion of health care reform has moved through time from some of the earliest philosophical ideas concerning the requisites for human flourishing to the introduction of utilitarianism in modern life, and its appropriation in the managerial search for cost-efficiency. Although we have not shared the same theoretical perspective, we have shared the commitment to an intellectual critique. What we have done in offering a number of different theoretical perspectives from our own portfolios of research is to make available to others what these positions have to offer in both understanding and explaining the phenomena of modern health care. The *complementary interpretations* of the subtitle refer to the value which each of us places on the different contribution of the other. The means whereby this process comes about is in the openness of dialogue and an eagerness to hear the contribution of one's colleagues; respecting and allowing the insights of others to refine and enrich our own.

Jane Robinson has treated policy as her empirical field of study. She has taken us through a detailed history of the values behind global initiatives aimed at improving the biological and economic health of some of the world's poorest countries. She has given an overview of the shifts in ascendant economic theories and political ideologies since the Second World War. For Jane, policy represents a set of practices with their own histories and discourses. Although policy is usually considered to be the instrument of change, Jane's approach to policy analysis challenges this view and argues that all policy embodies an inherent resistance to change, and a perpetuation of the status quo. The struggles on the part of institutions, national and international, governmental and local, to bring about effective and lasting improvements to health and health care can be seen in the context of this inherent resistance to change. Jane Robinson suggests that ongoing dialogue between the various competing interests offers the greatest hope for a sharing of insights into the complementary interpretations prevailing in modern health care, and the possibility (but no more) of making effective change.

Joanna Latimer draws on an anthropological approach to the practice–policy relation. In her ethnographic study of practice at the bedside of older people, Joanna shows the ways in which dominant relations are perpetuated. Joanna stresses how health needs are not givens, but matters of interpretation. Joanna emphasises how 'interests are connected to the ethical lives of social actors'. She examines the discursive practices of practitioners as they identify and name patients and their troubles, and lays these practices alongside practitioners' accounts of their practices and the policy context. She shows how practitioners draw on discourses, including those made available by policy, to accomplish the ordering of practice and their own identities. What emerges is how policy makes discursive positions available which practitioners can use to support a prevailing set of interests.

Mark Avis has explored notions of need and justice. Mark shows how the intellectual project is a process of continual dialogue in pursuit of an ethical base for the interpretation of need and the distribution of resources. Mark rejects the idea that the solution to these dilemmas can be solved by science alone, and reincorporates the eternal questions 'How should man live? and 'What is the good life?'. He uses philosophical procedures deriving from Wittgenstein and Winch to suggest an approach beyond relativism and foundationalism which allows different interpretations to come into play and to achieve an objective view of need and justice. This position allows the provisionality of truth and challenges practitioners to be continually reflective on their practice and the theoretical interpretations which underpin it.

Michael Traynor has examined the discursive practices of two groups, community nurses and senior NHS managers, generated by questionnaires concerned with job satisfaction, at staff meetings and in interviews. He shows that nurses and managers reach for readily available language and dualism to talk about themselves and each other, and to account for the value of their activities and their positions. Michael suggests that these discourses represent competing interests and are driven by potentially incommensurable values and objectives. He argues that underpinning these opposing views are different paradigms through which to constitute the purpose of health care and to interpret need and the allocation of resources.

So from the international policy-making of United Nations' agencies, to the individual nurse working in a client's home, no actor can avoid the powerful effect of a political, cultural and epistemological context. These changing contexts can be shaped by macro-economic factors, like the oil crises discussed by Jane Robinson, but without exception, they reach into the practices of all health workers. Similar effects can be found in the discourses of health policy aimed at reform across the globe. The support for new forms of financing for health care diminish previously powerful arguments that health care is unquestioningly a public good, and lead to the dilemmas epitomised by the poverty of care reported in some sub-Saharan African countries. 'Efficiency' and 'waste' and new forms of 'rationality', such as accounting technologies, have become powerful entities in the contemporary discourses of public policy.

In examining matters of interest in health policy and practice we have drawn on our different theoretical perspectives. All of these perspectives allow a provisionality of interpretation, none of which has claimed the dominance of a particular truth regime. By doing so we would merely have attempted to privilege one interpretative paradigm over another. Instead, we have recognised the contribution of each theoretical approach, and in entering into dialogue we have found that we occupy the spaces in between as each interacts with the other. It is our belief that models for good practice and policy in health care can be derived from a similar interaction of complementary interpretative positions that in themselves constitute the phenomenon of *interdisciplinarity*. We would go so far as to state that this is our hope for the future.

Index

A

Accountability, doctors' 168
Accounting technologies 166-167
Age, and social assessment 196–197
Anxiety, assessment of 201–202
Aristotle 94, 95, 102
Assessment
  by looking 200–204
  focus of 206
  of health needs 88–89
  and Maslow 86
  of patients 191–198
  and purchasing 138
  validity of 87
Astuteness, political 5
Autonomy
  nurses' 47, 143
  professional, and creation NHS 82
  as right 103
Awareness, political 5–7

B

Beds
  bed blocking strategies 173–174
  occupancy 171
  significance of term 191
Behaviour
  assessment of 200–202
  changing, and interests 165–166
Benefits
  economic 65–66
  health, definition 89
  social see social benefits
Bentham, Jeremy 108
Budget control
  see also finances
  by general practitioners 122
  and doctors 120–121
  and nurses 40
  and power 133–134
Bureaucracies, nature of 136
Bureaucrats, and nurses 151–153
Business, rationality 136–137

C

Canada, nursing in 6
Capabilities
  assessment of 203
  classification by 197–198
Care
  measurement by managers 127–132
  moral framework for 84
  and social status 23
Care systems, purpose 205
Caring
  and exploitation 153–154
  expression of 152–153
  and survival 145
Causality 192–193
Centralisation 121, 168
Changes, and reforms 36–37
Charity, and welfare 114
Chief Nurse Advisors 45–47
Church, NHS as 83
Civil liberties 111
Classification, of patients 198–200
Clay, Trevor 145–146
Clinical practice, responsibility for 167
Collectivism, and creation NHS 82
Colonialism, and development 68–69
Commitment, nurses' 154–155
Competition
  in NHS 120
  in World Bank policy 74, 75
Complaints, patients 169
Comprehensiveness, and creation NHS 82
Concerns see interests
Confidence, nurses' 6
Consensus management 38
Contracts, doctors 167
Control
  constructs 4–5
  of decision making 121
  of finances 134
  nurses 47
  and power 44
Critique
  intellectual 2
  and practice 4

Cultural artefacts, and identity 187
Culture
    and nursing 6
    of organisations 123–124
Culyer, A. 87–88

D

Dawkins, Richard 93
De Saussure, Ferdinand 147
Debt
    international
        repayment 53–54, 69
        and public health services 71
Decision making
    basis of nurses' 156–157
    by the public 138
    control of 121
    expression of 157–158
    and rationality 137–138
    responsibility for 38
    and utilitarianism 107
Decisions, legitimising 176–177, 178–179
Deconstruction, of nursing 1
Demand, for care, meeting 88
Deontology 155–156
Dependency
    and needs 82
    and poverty 76
Depression (1930's) 62
Descartes, René 11, 106
Desires, and needs 92
Development
    and colonialism 68–69
    and industrialisation 68–69
    and pluralism of ideas 73–74
Diagnosis 179–180
Difference principle 111, 112
Differences, and equality 102
Dilemmas, of intellectuals 3–4
Discharge, focus on 196–197, 205
Discipline, nurses 143–144
Discourses 90–91
    see also language
    analyses 149–150
    and power 136
Discretion, doctors' 168
Doctors
    see also health professionals
    accountability 168
    and budget control 120–121
    contracts 167
    discretion 168
    and efficiency 167
    and management 38–39

in management 120–121
power 46, 142
stereotypes 44, 142
Dualisms 141–142, 151–153
Duty
    and needs 102–103
    nurses' 153–154
    and rights 102–105
Duty of care 105–106, 116, 143
    and egalitarianism 112–113
    erosion of 180

E

Economic benefits 65–66
Economics
    engineering approach 59
    and ethics 58–59
    and health statistics 70
    and motivation 58, 59
    and social achievements 58
Economy, world, stabilisation 66–67
Education
    higher 5, 7
    multidisciplinary 7
    political 5–6
Efficiency
    and doctors 167
    and freedom of choice 68
    monitoring 41, 42
    and practice 34
    and utilitarianism 58
    and World Bank policy 75
Egalitarian theory, of social justice
        110–113
Egyptian Sanitary Maritime and
        Quarantine Board 61
Engineering approach, to economics 59
Enlightenment project 11–12
Entitlement theory, of social justice
        113–114
Epidemiology, and health needs
        assessment 89
Equality 100–102
Equity
    approach to policy 58
    and creation NHS 82
    and Quality Adjusted Life Years
        109–110
    in WHO and UNICEF policies 70
    and World Health Organization 62
Ethics
    and economics 58–59
    of health care 180
    and needs 81

and research 24
and tensions 4
Examination, purpose of 190
Excellence 115
Exclusion
    at bedside 172–180
    patient, justification for 205–206
Expertise, and research outcome 34
Experts, and goals 87
Exploitation 157
    and caring 153–154

F

Fair opportunity 112
Family, responsibility for care 205
Feasibility, strategies 63–64
Finances
    see also budget control
    awareness in NHS 166–167
    control by Trusts 122
    management by doctors 120–121
    and morals 158
    and tensions 4
Financial rationality 132–135
Foucault, Michel 90
    and medicine 189–190
Freedom 59
    of choice, and efficiency 68
    and USA policies 68
    and World Health Organization 62
Function, and genes 93–94

G

Garage, NHS as 83
Gaze
    nursing 200–204
    professional 189–191
Gender
    see also women
    and health care 73
    and occupations 45
General Practitioner fundholders 122
Genes, and function 93–94
Goals
    of care, identifying 197–199
    and experts 87
    and individuality 88
    and morals 114–115
    and needs 84–85, 87–88
    and teleology 93
Governmentality effect 168
Governments

and public health 65
    spending priorities 77
Great Britain, policy rationale 75
Griffiths enquiry 33–34
Griffiths and the Nurses 46
Griffiths reforms 37–41

H

Health
    health benefit 89
    health economists, and needs 87–88
    and international financial
        institutions 56–57
    needs assessment 88–89
    policy, and needs 58
    and poverty 74
    as right 103
    statistics, and economic policies 70
'Health for all' 61–62, 72
Health of the Nation strategy 72
Health professionals
    effect of reforms on 36–37
    role 55, 83–84
    and service provision 88–89
Human flourishing 94, 95–96, 115
    and policy 77

I

Ideas, plurality of 72–75
Identity
    and interests 204–207
    and performance 187–189
    transforming 176–178
Ignorance 111–112, 116–117
Image, post Griffiths 48
Impartiality 101–102
Individualism, and social justice
        114–115
Individuals
    and goals 88
    in utilitarianism 106–107
Industrialisation, and development
        68–69
Information, Chief Nurse Advisors'
        access to 47
Information systems 41
Information Technology, use in
        measurement 129–130, 132
Insurance, health 74
Intellectuals
    dilemmas of 3–4
    role of 2–3

Interests 164–166
   and behaviour 165–166
   competing 49–50
   and identity 187–188, 204–207
   reconstructing 36
Internal market 121–122
International Bank for Reconstruction
      and Development 62
   see also World Bank
International Development
      Association 62
International Finance Corporation 63
International financial institutions, and
      health 56–57
International health policy, eras of 60
International Monetary Fund
   policies 60
   and health care 71–72
International organisations
   influencing health policy 61–63
   viability 64
International Sanitary Conference, Paris
      1851, 65
Investing in Health 74–75
Issues, legitimacy 63

J

Judgement, and resistance 156–157

K

Knowledge
   downgrading professionals' 137
   and feasibility 64
   language 127
   magnifying 174–175
   objective knowledge 10–15
   valid 128–129
Kuhn, Thomas 13

L

Language
   see also discourses
   importance of 15–16
   and knowledge 127
   and management 123
   of need 84–85
   and power 136–137
   of rights 103
   and structuralism 146–147
   use by managers 135, 136, 137

Leadership, post Griffiths 43
League of Nations 61, 67
Legitimacy, issues 63
Libertarian theory, of social justice 113–114
Liberty principle 111, 112
Looking, as assessment 200–204

M

MacIntyre, Alasdair 94–95, 114–115
   and managers 124
   and manipulation 135–136
Management
   by doctors 120–121
   effect of reforms on 36–37
   and information 127–132
   introduction to NHS 37–41
   and language 123
   and performance 123, 124
   responsibility pre Griffiths 38–39
Managerialism 123–124
   and nursing 145–146
Managers
   and information 127–132
   and measurement 127–132
Manipulation
   by managers 135–136
   of needs 107
Market economy, and libertarianism
      113–114
Markets
   and authority 133–134
   in NHS 120
Maslow 85–86
Measurement
   by managers 127–132
   of care 127–132
   privileging of 137
   and uncertainty 137–138
Medicine
   discipline of 189–191
   as managing 205
   rationality of 136–137
Metaphor management 135, 137
Minorities, position of 2
Mobility, focus on 195, 197, 205
Morality
   and nursing 142–145
   of nursing 154–155, 157
Morals
   and finances 158
   frameworks for care 84
   and goals 114–115
   moral discourse 153
   moral purposes 94–95

Morals (*contd*)
    and needs 85, 86, 88, 103
    and social justice 115
    and utilitarianism 106, 107
Motivation, and economics 58, 59
Mutual aid, in NHS 83

N

National Health Service
    in 1970's 166–168
    in 1980's 166–168
    and needs 82–92
    NHS and Community Care
        Act 1990, 121
    policy objectives, and social
        justice 106
    principles underpinning creation 82
    public perception 166–168
    reforms 35–37, 119, 121–122
    social purpose 83
    strains on 166–168
Need
    grammar of 84
    nature of 84–85
Needs
    assessment 88–89
    being instrumental 86–87
    and dependency 82
    and desires 92
    and duty 102–103
    and egalitarianism 112–113
    and ethics 81
    and goals 84–85
    health care, definition 89
    and health economists 87–88
    and morals 85, 86, 88, 103
    and the NHS 82–92
    nurses perception of 86–87, 155–156
    and objectivity 84, 87, 92–96
    and obligation 84
    and policy 58, 81–82, 83
    and psychological states 92–93
    relativity of 85
    social justice perspectives 102, 116
    as universal drives 85–86, 93–94
    visibility 105–106
NHS and Community Care Act 1990, 121
Nozick, R. 113
Numbers, in measurement 127–130
Nurses
    see also health professionals
    autonomy 143
    and budget control 40
    and bureaucrats 151–153

Chief Nurse Advisors 45–47
    identity 193–194
    and information collection 129, 130
    legitimising practice 206–207
    as managers 42–43
    Nurse Executive Directors 121
    nurse leaders 43, 45–47, 121
    perception of need 86–87
    power 142–143, 156, 159–160
    recruitment 44
    registration 144
    response to Griffiths report 39
    role 104–105
    and sacrifice 142–145, 157–158
    stereotypes 44, 142–143
    values 86, 146, 152–155
Nursing
    deconstruction of 1
    expertise 200–204
    management post Griffiths 39
    and managerialism 145–146
    organisation 49
    rationality of 136–137
Nursing Policy Studies Centre 34

O

Objectivity 10–15
    and needs 84, 95–96
    predominance of 137–138
    rediscovering objective needs 92–96
    use of 91–92
Obligation, and needs 84
Occupations, and gender 45
Office International d'Hygiene Publique
        61, 67
Older people
    classification of 171–172
    concerns of 187–188
    discourses about 170–172, 191–194
    social assessment 196–197
Opportunities, and liberty 112
Opportunity costs 99–100
    visibility of 105
Organisations
    culture 123–124
    nursing 49
Our Common Future 73
Outcomes, and quality 167

P

Pan American Sanitary Bureau 61, 67
Patients
    classifying 170

excluding from care 172–180
as management targets 170–172
responsibility for care 205
Patient's Charter 168–169
Pea lady 174–179
Performance
and identity 187–189
and management 123, 124
and throughput 163–164
Philosophers, postmodernist 12–16
Philosophy, and nursing 9–16
Policy
basis for 88
economic benefits 65–66
and health practitioners' role 55
international, post second world war
67–69
and needs 82, 83
process 63–67
and resources 88
utilitarian approach 58, 107
Politics
nurses' awareness 5–7
and public health 65–66
Postmodernists 12–13, 89–92
Poststructuralism 148–149
Poverty
and dependency 76
and health 74
and structural adjustment 74
Power
and behaviour 20
and budget control 40
Chief Nurse Advisors 47
constructs 4–5
and control 44
and discourse 90
doctors 46, 142
and language 136–137
nurses' 156, 159–160
Practice
and critique 4
and efficiency 34
Preference–satisfaction 106–109
Priestley, Clive 37–38
Privatisation 75
Professionals, identity 188–189, 190
Psychological states, and needs
92–93
Public, and decision making 138
Public health
and governments 65
and political interests 65–66
and scientific evidence 67
Purchasing, and assessment 138
Purpose, care systems 205

Q

Quality
of care 154
clinical practice 167
criteria of 156–157
monitoring 41, 42
Quality Adjusted Life Years 109–110

R

Rationalism, of managers 159–160
Rationality, and decision making
137–138
Rawls, John 111–113, 115, 116–117
Reality, discovering 10–11
Recession, 1970's 69–72
Recruits, to nursing 44
Reform weariness 37
Reforms
and changes 36–37
Griffiths 37–41
health care, 1990's 75
National Health Service 35–37, 119
significant 35–36
Registration, nurses 144
Relativity, of needs 85
Research
and ethics 24
and practice changes 25
Research outcome, and expertise 34
Resistance, and judgement 156–157
Resources
see also social benefits
allocation 99–100
for caring 154
and entitlement theory 113
and equality 101
and policy 88
and utilitarianism 110
Responsibility, in NHS 83
Rhetoric, of managers 127, 135
Rights 59
and duties 102–105
and equality 100–101
in language 103
negative rights 103
positive rights 103–104
right to assistance 104
social justice perspectives 116
to care 155–156
and utilitarianism 108, 110
Rorty, Richard 12–14, 15
Royal College of Nursing research,
impact 1991 reforms 150–160

S

Sacrifice, and time 157–158
Said, Edward 2
Sceptics 11
Science, and knowledge 11–14
Scientific evidence, and public health 67
Self sacrifice, and nursing 142–145
Selfish gene theory 93
Semiotics 146–147
Sen, Amartya 58–59, 94–95
Services, supply 88–89
Signs
    of activity 203
    in language 147, 148–149
    of problems 195–196
Social achievements, and economics 58
Social artefacts, and identity 187
Social benefits
    see also resources
    distribution 108
    prioritising distribution 111
Social class, and nursing 6–7
Social contract 111–113
Social influences, health 89
Social justice
    approach to policy 58
    and equality 100–102
    explanation 100
    and morals 115
    theories of 106–114
    in WHO and UNICEF policies 70
    and World Health Organization 62
Social situation, nurses concern with
        194–198
Social status, and care 23
Socialism, and health care policy 69
Society, participation 95–96
Strains, on health care systems 166–168
Strategies, feasibility 63–64
Structural adjustment 71–72, 73
Structuralism 148–149
    and language 146–147
Subjectivity, and desire 84
Submissiveness, of nursing 142–143
Surveillance 137
    of nurses 143–144
Surveys, patient satisfaction 169
Survival, and needs 93–94
Sustainability 76

T

Teleology
    and biology 93–94

and moral purposes 94–95
Tensions
    and ethics 4
    sources 4
Throughput
    and health issues 205
    nurses alignment on 205–206
    and performance 163–164
    requirements for 205–206
    as strategic value 168–170
    strategies promoting 173–174
Time
    for caring 154
    and sacrifice 157–158
    and throughput 168–169
Training 70–71, 154–155
Trusts, NHS 122

U

United Nations, origins 61
United Nations Conference on
        International Organisation
        61–62
United States of America
    nursing in 6
    and United Nations policy 67–68
Universal drives, and needs 85–86
Universality, and creation NHS 82
Utilitarianism 106–110
    in nursing 159–160
    and policy 58
Utility
    explanation 106–107
    and Quality Adjusted Life Years
        109–110

V

Values
    nurses' 86, 146, 152–155
    throughput 168–170
Vocation, nurses' 153–155

W

Ward design, and discipline 143–144
Welfare
    and charity 114
    discourse 155
Women
    see also gender
    and nursing's status 143, 144
    responsibility for care 205
    and tradition 137

Working for Patients 121–122
  Royal College of Nursing's view
    145–146
World Bank
  objectives 56, 66
  origins 61, 62–63
  policies 56, 59–60, 73–75
  working with World Health
    Organization 74
World Commission on Environment and
  Development 73

World Health Organization
  objectives 66–67
  origins 61–62, 63
  policies 59, 72–73
  working with World Bank 74

Z

Zambia, health in 53, 54